Unparalleled
Sorrow

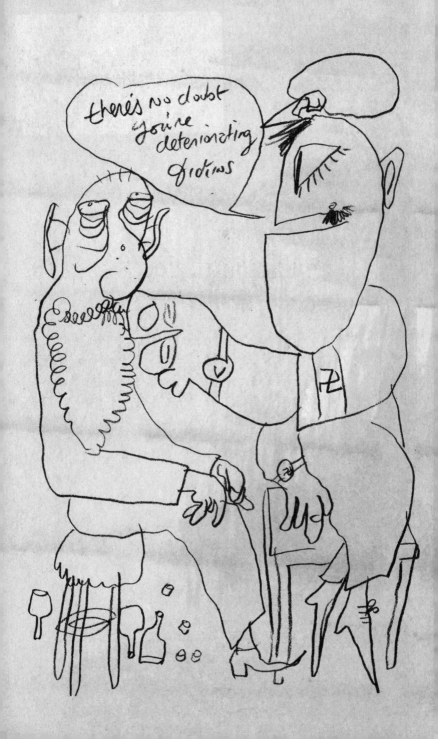

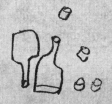

Unparalleled
Sorrow

*Finding my way
back from
depression*

Barry Dickins

hardie grant books

*Dedicated to Tom Gelai, who never judged me or felt
sorry for me when I was in that wretched clinic
on and off for six awful months.*

Published in Australia in 2009 by
Hardie Grant Books
85 High Street
Prahran, Victoria 3181, Australia
www.hardiegrant.com.au

The moral rights of the author have been asserted.
Copyright © Barry Dickins 2009

A catalogue record for this book is available from the National Library of Australia.
ISBN: 9781740668033

Cover and text design by Michelle Mackintosh
Illustrations by Barry Dickins
Printed and bound in Australia by McPherson's Printing Group

10 9 8 7 6 5 4 3 2 1

The names of some people and places have been changed for legal reasons.

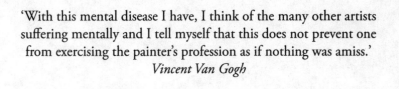

'With this mental disease I have, I think of the many other artists suffering mentally and I tell myself that this does not prevent one from exercising the painter's profession as if nothing was amiss.'
Vincent Van Gogh

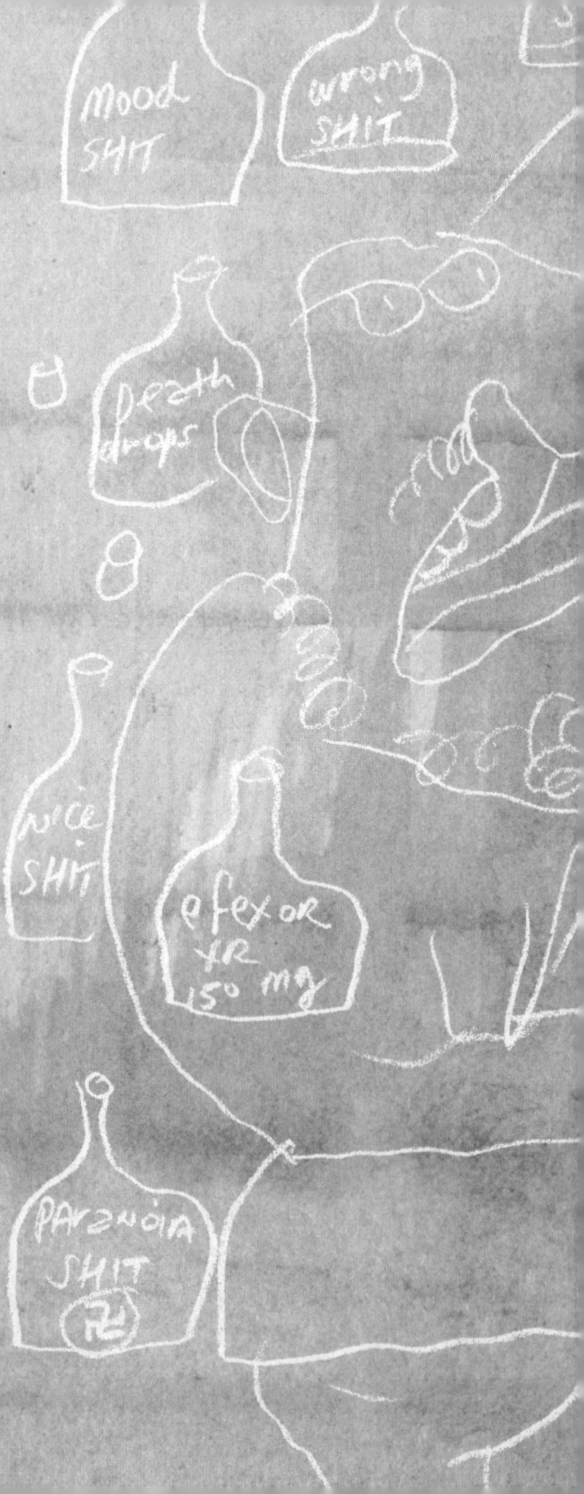
mood SHIT
wrong SHIT
Death drops
nice SHIT
efexor XR 150 mg
Paranoia SHIT

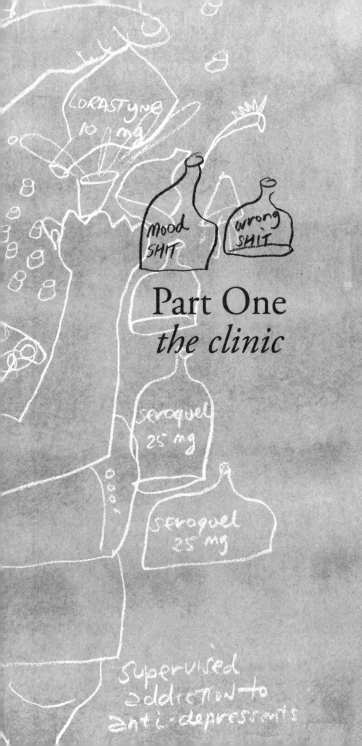

Part One
the clinic

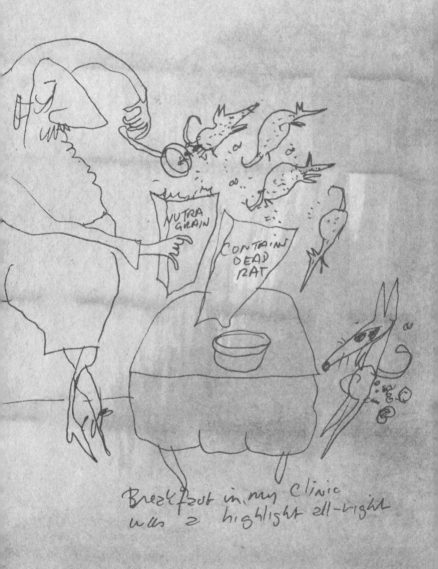

NUTRA GRAIN

CONTAINS DEAD RAT

Breakfast in my clinic was a highlight all-right

Chapter
one

I CAN'T REMEMBER going to bed the night before my first ECT. Or giving my permission or my wife giving her consent, but she and my brother Chris did and for my part I was so confused I would've agreed to be shot at point-blank range by a firing squad. Try as I might I couldn't get comfortable that night; I remember the physical distress and the floating stomach and wriggling and rubbing and twitching of my feet in bed before they came to collect me at 6 am exactly.

I was pretty paranoid and four silhouetted nurses were right by the bed. My room felt like it had humanly betrayed me in sleep, the sleep of reason. Soon I would be given a shot of electricity to lift my mood, as they kept putting it. What on earth is so wrong with sadness? My wife was my dearest friend but has decided to split and prefers to live alone. 'I'm very sorry but I don't love you anymore.' That handwritten death sentence of hers kept on echoing in my subconscious as one big dark nurse held a torch in the dimness of early ghastly morning. Must they be to be so melodramatic? Why didn't we just walk off to the Recovery Room as friends together without the vigilante feeling?

I recognised just who they were now and they came into sore-eyed focus as I put my black velveteen pants on with the long dumb vinyl belt – I'd lost a kilo since I arrived at the mental hospital not far from the city and that felt good as I was much too heavy before – so I put on my black vinyl carpet slippers and dark blue cotton top and one of them beckoned me to follow them as they got in close to me and we walked quickly to the pinging elevator.

Some of the patients' doors were left wide open and they were either out like a light or merely sitting there on the edge of perfect anonymity, just agape with woe or smiling at nothing. The squad of really fit nurses put me into a chromium and steel enormous squat lift that made no sound at all as its thick big door opened to suck us all into it and down to the Recovery Room. None of the nurses said anything of comfort such as, 'This will lift your mood' or 'You'll recover much quicker after ECT'; they just looked morosely at me as I stared in an uneasy way at four or five unconscious bodies who'd just been given it.

They really resembled Caucasian corpses and had dull, uncleaned, yellowish teeth with their arms hanging down or folded up or any old way: old depressives all put out to it and tongues hanging out in dumbness like the great dumbness of animals, except they didn't have the nobility. Some were beginning to rouse and one had awoken and had a tartan green and red dressing-gown wrapped round him; he put his reading spectacles on and sat up and, in his white jocks, got in his wheelchair and a female nurse chatted with him in a bubbly familiar manner as she quickly wheeled him towards the surreal lift. He's a Collins Street businessman, well known in finance.

There was a nurse, Ian, dabbing conductive on a lady's white blank forehead and she held his palm for the security, which of course Ian loved, and then she had to lie perfectly flat on the theatre bed, which had a white sheet stretched tight over it, and a nurse dabbed the conductive gel upon her hair a bit now and put the electricity tapes on the nape of her old neck and gave her a short square anaesthetic needle speedily and accurately and then held a yellowish transparent gas mask over her open mouth and she was gassed.

She was oblivious now and her body was very stiff indeed and the nurses conversed to her unconsciousness as she was administered a jolt of current to lift her mood, as they kept on putting it. That's all they could say here. It's enough to depress you. After ten minutes she came to and was wheeled away back to bed and another person hopped on the bed for his go.

I was sitting very uncomfortably within a great big dark pink floral armchair, which was the most awkward object I'd ever sat in, and I stared within sleepiness at the others either being given it or coming out of it. This was not Jack Nicholson in *One Flew Over the Cuckoo's Nest* but Barry Dickins being electrocuted to bring me back to normality.

A big letterbox-mouth nurse uncurled his forefinger to me, meaning 'next'; everything is pantomime here, and like a child I reluctantly got on the hard ECT bench and gazed up at them helplessly. They were all upside-down-looking and one lady nurse had appalling body odour. Maybe her odour that was so fetid would lift my mood to a greater clinical depression? I could go right off the scale soon.

I felt like I was in a short scene from a television hospital drama but it was all perfectly real. They leant over me in face masks and rapidly, without any explanation, dabbed the electricity gel on my mousy sticky-up hair I'd never been able to do a thing with; it always goes its own stubborn anti-gravity way, and now they nimbly applied the tapes with little adhesive tabs on my neck and gave me the needle and I really jerked when they forced the plastic gas mask on my dry mouth. I wanted to be sick.

'Take one or two really big breaths, Barry, now and just try and relax,' whispered one of them, holding me down very flat, as I was trying really hard to get up. I showed no initiative and breathed in the revolting gas, which smelt shocking. My racing memory remembered instinctively being given chloroform when I was about six years old at the Royal Children's Hospital; it still lingers persistently in my spirit, which is human memory. I hoped I wouldn't lose it.

The deep gulps of breath over, I was felled like a morose seal being innoculated with a drug-dart and my heavy 58-year-old head fell right on my chest and I was unavailable for comment. I couldn't feel the current going through me or sense anything at all as I was assisted into the wheelchair and they put a blanket over me and ran me like anything to the sinister lift, the sneering inhuman lift, to rush me back to Room 5, my crypt. Did the nurses all not laugh as they *ran* me?

I felt violated and remorseful and numb and nauseous as they prised me into bed. Sharna, the nurse, materialised. 'Did you sleep in your clothes last night? Didn't you bother to put on your pyjamas? You are slack!' My old dry moisture-seeking tongue wanted sparkling lemonade on it. The conductive gel felt slimy in my greasy hair on the pillow. I was all so slimey – yuk!

The stress of the first ECT had given me bad heartburn so my chest pained me and I required Quik-Eze indigestion lollies, but they had none of those at the hospital. 'All you do today after your first ECT, Mr Dickins, is sleep,' one of them cautioned me. They departed and I was instructed to lie there and simply relax, but that isn't as easy as it sounds. Why did I give my permission, why did my wife? It was foolish. What had they done? I picked up a piece of paper and a fine-liner and put it on my knee and tried to print my own name but it was nervous scribble and my fingertips vibrated so I couldn't hold it still. What if I could never draw again? Or write with my pen or pencil as I had all my life so far?

I felt damned to hell and that's not an over-statement but a simple fact. I kept running my hands through where they put the conductive gel and I kept on jerking around and wriggling, like a sort of dance routine in my bed; I couldn't lie still after it. I was just shaking.

Outside, not far from the city, it was raining and the unminding rain struck my big window pane and I could faintly detect frantic public servants running back to their computers, holding wet newspapers over their wet heads after their lunch break was over and giggling girls running in stiletto heels and parking officers having their fun booking motorists for being on the road. People eating hurried sandwiches on their break, people coughing, getting on the crowded city tram, people hurrying back from the hairdresser, all the tiny dramas of ordinary existence that I had captured in my writing, in my newspaper columns, in my books of essays, the love of the everyday. Everyman. I go for Everyman.

But would ECT lift my mood? How could it change my divorce coming up? Wouldn't it contribute? How many times will I be given a dose? Once? A hundred?

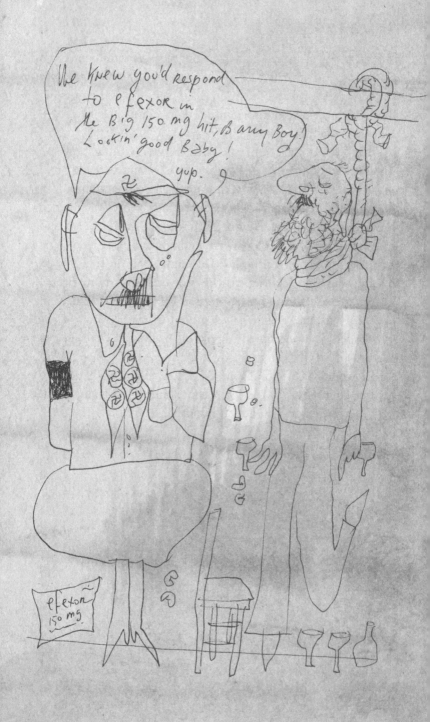

Chapter
two

THE CLINIC IS where I have been admitted today and given an awful room immediately and had my underpants inserted in the bottom drawer and my socks in there too. They sent me over here from St Vincent's Hospital in Nicholson Street, where my wife escorted me in a state of bewilderment, my speech slurred and slowed right down to a hoarse impersonation of my old faithful voice, the voice of a comedian. I have joked and talked briskly all my life and that life has been spent in the street with the continuously comical tragic interrupting voices I have heard and stored up and revised and redrafted as theatre scripts and ABC Radio plays recorded in Sydney and Melbourne and Adelaide. I am fifty-eight and have given my life to popular entertainment: satirical columns in newspapers and stand-up comedy in pubs. I'm an artist. A licorice allsort.

What led me to St Vincent's to be mentally assessed was continuous insomnia, caused by loud insectish noises in my head called tinnitus that robbed me of sleep and drove me just about mad. The neverending whistling of tinnitus is pretty much unbearable; my old mother has had it since she had her first breakdown forty years ago, so she, poor creature, just stares at the darkened blinds all night in her childish bedroom with big dolls on the bed. A little girl at eighty-five. Poor thing: I love her so much.

My tinnitus got worse twenty years ago by living in Separation Street, Northcote, with my wife right on the main road with deafening trucks roaring through from dawn till dark and cars starting up, it seemed, right inside your pillow. I dropped sleeping pills but I had to gulp a lot of them to get completely out to it, and then the traffic woke me up anyway so I went without sleep altogether, often drinking wine in the day to relax and chainsmoking to wind down from the tension. I became a drunk. At least that was easy. I didn't have to try hard to do that. And wrote hung over and taught class hung over and made love hung over, which contributed to the destruction of my marriage. It's all my fault.

At St Vincent's they told me there could be permanent brain damage. I didn't feel permanently brain damaged. I felt the same way, whatever that was. Just me. The same me as yesterday. But they stared critically at me and were sure there was damage. In the end I tended to agree with them. I must have been damaged if I felt this bad. Panicking and thinking of the worst possible outcome, almost hallucinatory. You're right; I'm mad. I think we all shook hands.

It all started back in March last year on an author's tour of a little town named Wangaratta when I became unwell, and one thing led to another before the complete cave-in physically and mentally. The library in Wangaratta wrote to me offering a residency of country libraries to read from my books to audiences out of touch with city writers. Obscure people in obscure places: some would be in mobile caravans and possibly paddocks where I'd read to them in my hopefully winning way from a deckchair. The pay was good, two hundred bucks a library and motel chucked in. In fact it was a very agreeable arrangement indeed especially for the thirty books I'd had published; it would boost their popularity. Bring them back into print.

I'm a pretty good reader-aloud from my work and have performed heaps of live readings in libraries and pubs and schools and TAFES and every possible venue since I was first published many decades ago; it is a thing I adore to do so I wrote back to say okay and the next thing I'm driving up to Wang. In the 1990 white Corolla sedan.

The gig was for five days so I would come home with a thousand bucks. I had been finding sleep hard to come by due to the tinnitus, which was getting worse and much louder and more penetrating than ever, like an infernal whistle down in my ear canal that demented me with its conniving persistence. The prescription sleeping capsules just didn't work.

I used to like getting stuck in heavy traffic because with all the engines roaring away I actually couldn't hear my own tinnitus sawing my nerves away like a bandsaw. I rejoiced in coagulated traffic and must have been the only motorist in Melbourne who avoided a clear run. I adored tunnels best because of the fumes and the pitch of whining motorbikes and gargling semi-trailers all chomping each other right up.

Anyway, here I was pulling into dear Wangaratta and the Corolla went okay and I felt pretty good although my wife and I had been fighting a lot lately and sleeping apart. Or being sleepless apart. I'm impossible to live with. Or be alone with.

I noticed my fingers were shaking as I signed in at reception and that my famous handwriting was a bit spidery, a bit jumpy, as was my voice when the motel lady asked me if I wanted Coco Pops to take back to my room with a copy of *The Age*. I could not compute. I didn't know why I was actually doing this.

It was about six at night and I had a hot bath, lucky to score a tub. I shampooed the outer self. I dried my fuzzy mousey hair and draped on fresh clothes and went for a stroll around town. Folks were out walking and the town hall clock gonged away and kids were on bikes and skateboards and there were the usual archetypes, stalkers, rapists, librarians. I didn't know whether I was hungry or not and hit my pocket to make sure I had enough change for a cheeseburger and a thickshake because I remembered that they made pretty decent strawberry thickshakes in Wang. The very best.

My mind was all over the place but I never worried too much about that because it had happened since I was a manic-depressed infant; the moods swinging up and down like a cerebral pendulum within me and without drugs; there's nothing one can do but put up with the highs and lows that arrive and depart upon the instant. It's so tiring. I sort of wanted to talk to people but sort of didn't because I really didn't want to annoy anybody, especially in Wang as they all looked pretty annoyed anyway; they all had a put-out look or was that my imagination? Possibly. My imagination exhausts me.

I came home to my temporary oasis, the sterile motel where the man at reception asked me why I was there, and I replied that I was an author on an author's tour of country libraries and then he laughed.

Whatever on earth was funny about that? I went to my room and ate a few pears I brought up from Melbourne with me and watched a bit of ultra-violent American trash on the overhead telly and thought about which particular books I would read from the next morning. But there wasn't anything on in the morning; it wasn't until night right here in Wang and then as I studied the printed schedule of my readings I started to become anxious that I'd got all the dates wrong. In fact, everything was wrong.

I sat on the edge of the hard, uncosy motel bed and kept on reading the program over and over through my spectacles, the pair I sat on; luckily, I had a back-up pair in the glovebox of the Corolla. Then I realised I had to go to Wangaratta Library at ten the next day to meet the staff and discuss the tour. I had to perform at Bright and Myrtleford and off-the-map country towns with only beauty and sheep in them.

I heard guests next door arguing gently. Cars arriving noisily and people playing loud music and trucks and doors slamming like loud heartbeats. I went out and bought a burger and sipped a cup of tea, white one sugar, and sat in the warm March moonlight remembering the abstract quarrels with my wife; I couldn't recall what they were about though, usually she called me 'such a bully' and slammed doors. Maybe it had to do with her not wanting sex with me anymore. Or the abandonment of the physical altogether as one falls out of love after twenty-seven years, and there is no touching, only touchiness. I love her. Do I?

Prickliness so there were no quiet moments nor restful seconds unless the telly was on and I had begun to detest all television and become bored with whatever moronic show was on. Why did we stay together when it was so obviously hopeless? She toiled from early till late as a Catholic primary school teacher and had rheumatism and had ordered a hip replacement for Christmas. She'd already gone through her change of life, the end of the menstrual cycle, but she seemed bad-tempered to me; possibly it was my fault she's having a hip replacement. We were once such good friends when we met by chance in 1982.

I remembered the decent reviews for some of my books and the awards I'd scored over the years, including the Victorian Premiers Award for Drama in 1994 and the International Amnesty Award for Peace through Art for my stage play *Remember Ronald Ryan*, which looked behind the headlines at the real story of our country's last executed person. I couldn't have written about execution after our only baby was born in 1995.

Cases of my books and cases of my public successes mixed

with the crumple of my marriage is not the way towards a good night's sleep before a reading and in the darkness of the awfully stuffy motel room, with its heady aroma of loneliness of the spirit and surgical carpet and plastic dustmotes I kept on seeing my wife's teeth meeting and forming the sentence, 'I'm very sorry but I don't love you anymore.'

She's not being hateful when she says things like that; I'm sure I'm hard to live with but we've had a lot of fun over the decades we've been together, then having the baby so late, she at forty-two and me at forty-six, and how dangerously sick she was when the baby came due to pre-eclampsia, the blackness of her face and the horror in her eyes and me snipping the cord through a rainfall of grateful sobs.

Why do we fight so much lately? It's my drinking. But I don't always drink. The white wine out in the miniature courtyard, the staring up at the heavens for clues to my self-indulgent existence, drinking stubbies later as my son and tired wife flake out after a tough day at their schools and more plonk as I serve up. The predictable scorched sausages took all gloss off the fun. I was never shown how to cook. Never how to clean.

She has always been cautious with her alcoholic consumption and I've only ever seen her drunk twice in all the years we've been married, once after a pub crawl in the city and once after a particularly dull party when she drank out of boredom. Again the hallucinatory teeth revolve in thin motel air and form the gruelling sentence that goes, 'I'm terribly sorry but I'm afraid I don't love you anymore.' No wonder she doesn't. Who could? Not me.

I have been hung over driving my happy little boy to his grammar school in South Yarra, driving pretty safely but nevertheless not the best and apprehensive about big trucks on Hoddle Street and how light our car is, and that it wouldn't take much to die.

This was the incorrect method of gaining repose and I just thrashed about all night, full of Coco Pops and sleeping capsules; I got up buggered the next morning to meet the Wang Librarian and walked there. That was enjoyable; it always is, walking after a rotten motel night with no sleep in it.

I was greeted and spoke confidently, pretty much, but felt so strange, like some sort of gloomy circus mallet kept hitting me on the head. I was introduced to a woman mobile-van driver who looked Amazonian. She had impressive biceps and was an effortless raconteur and a safe driver and it felt terrific to be out in the backblocks and looking at the bush, bulls and what have you. You know how the bush is: pretty barren and suicidal. Do bulls take their own lives?

We arrived at a bush hut or something with a few old former church chairs or pews in it and she set up the books on tables for bush women to choose from, or bush gentlemen with carefully polished reading spectacles over their proboscises and I went for a stroll through the paddocks to sip in the gorgeous mountain air. That old good-to-be-alive sensation came back again, and she handed me a big black Nescafé heaped with white sugar for the necessary lift in mood.

Maybe she could tell how anxious I was becoming, I could feel the panic rise up in my being; it's illogical but there it is, the fear of being in public to speak, which is the best thing I'm capable of, that's me at my best. I'm a great reader but felt terrible, dry-mouthed and aching in the shoulders and stiff in the neck and just needing to sleep.

To my astonishment she didn't remember to pack any of my books. Not one of them and there are nearly thirty all up over the years, plays and fiction and anthologies of remembrance and books of my poetry and children's picture books. No books!

So I had to tell the ladies and old codgers sitting in this hut in a paddock how I went about creating my most popular children's picture book, entitled *My Grandmother*, back in 1988 for Penguin, doing all the pen and ink drawings and the watercolour wrap-around cover artwork. It would have been so much more reassuring to read from the actual published book instead of nervously reminiscing like this. I was falling apart at the seams here in a paddock!

So I just pulled my chair near the bush book borrowers in that strange hut in the strange paddock with the kangaroos all through it and remembered my grandmother to them, hundreds of embroidered anecdotes all sewn together and how she lived to be a day off a hundred and made the decision to die by starving herself to death, but I leavened it with lots of light-heartedness and in fact I gave good hut. I needed to wee after a two-hour talk but there was no loo. I considered urinating in the splendid paddock but some of them would no doubt have seen me so I just had to bloody well hang on till Wang. No books and she's the driver for the Wang mobile books.

It was early afternoon when we returned so I had an unsuccessful rest on the motel bed trying to be unconscious until the night reading at the big Wang Library at 8 pm. More no-use sleeping tablets and I was unable to chew my bread correctly because the horrid stone-ground bread rolls stuck irremovably to my fibreglass dentures. I just sipped soda water all day but that made me rapidly urinate; it always does. I'm a fool, a near perfect fool, you'd have to say. I would have swapped my immortal soul for half an hour's sleep, no problem. You go mad when you can't get any.

About six o'clock I bought myself a piece of fried flake and a minimum of fatty chips and wondered why it was I developed chronic heartburn straight away as I sat eating it in a park with pederasts dotted all through it. I made the considerable error of swallowing a giant takeaway black coffee with six sugars in it to try to pep myself up for the concert in half an hour; there was a big audience when I went in and a big photo of me when I was much younger, taken from the newspaper maybe thirty years before to support one of my columns.

MEET BARRY DICKINS LIVE said the banner. Well, that is something I want to do, I thought to myself as I headed to the desk where they had me set up without a microphone or a jug of iced water. Some old lady introduced me as Australia's funniest man. Am I? Was I?

My palms were all sweaty and I couldn't stop writhing in my chair. My old throat was so dry and I could feel newly formed half-inch-wide mouth ulcers in my mouth due to eating no fruit; was that it? I needed to die. That's best when you're reduced to this.

I started off with the usual palaver of wafting from the working classes and being a poor, disinterested student at school and falling in love with poetry at the tender age of ten and surrendering to literature all my life, and they seemed to be liking what I was saying but then someone just called out, 'Speak up' and I didn't know what that meant so I ignored that rudeness and just kept on speaking in exactly the same way, with a soft, intimate and winning tone. I was two feet away from the microphone, which actually *was* there.

I was used to being fascinating. The library patrons couldn't hear me. At least they had a few of my old books on display, so that felt pretty helpful. The problem was I was completely distracted by everything I looked at, especially them, the people who looked like studies out of Hieronymous Bosch sketchbooks, who'd come along to see me and hear me read in my winning way, with loads of extemporisations thrown in for good measure.

My family was breaking up and so was my heart, banging away so loudly I assumed the audience could hear it tom-tomming away. I couldn't adjust my countenance from death to life, my lips refused to smile, though I very much felt like genuinely smiling at them and putting on a good show. I'm a showman. One old man showed me his handwritten novel that took him ten years to write after his wife left him after sixty years of faithful marriage. I asked him if he had a photocopy and he said he didn't and looked down in a flat way at his shoes. I put him off. I depressed him more than his 100-year-old missus leaving him.

The lonely expression in his old eyes really got to me and I reluctantly plucked up his manila folder with its hundreds of pages crammed into it with ultrafine spidery hand writing all through it, single-spaced of course; it was tragic he told me, a tragic family saga and he confessed no one had read it before and he'd always treasured my style and had kept toffee-coloured, tatty old cuttings of my *Sun News Pictorial* columns in scrapbooks he'd patiently clagged in over decades of studying me in print. I just couldn't handle him. I hated him.

I did my level best but it wasn't good enough to be called professional. The library girl who served the refreshments had said I was unwell before my talk started; she stressed this. I suppose she could tell my health was bad in one glance. I usually press the flesh after an engagement and sit round listening to country people talk about sheep drench and when the fox got the cocky in its cage, stuff like that. And folks were kind of relaxing with me and sipping their teas and coffees and munching a few homemade muffins and talking accurately and grimly about climate change, about which I knew nothing. But after an hour and a half I blankly shook hands with the friendly staff and after being given a navy blue paper serviette containing muffins for the motel, I walked home feeling perfectly hollow. I was nothing. I had no feeling. A void. I was clichéd.

I wasn't hungry, not even peckish, and all the words in the daily newspaper swam, and I swam round the room mentally with my wife's declaration of our ending just being spoken by her repeatedly; the millions of things we'd done together were in the crowded room with me and the bric-a-brac and antiques we'd saved for or bought on impulse, the furniture we'd lay-byed together was in the room, everything was in the room. I couldn't blame her, only my illness, which wore her right out.

I knew I was to live with my son and drive him to school and she was to renovate our terrace and live alone in it. Rent out a room. Everything seemed meaningless. Except the memory of our boy being born thirteen years before; I could hear his contagious laughter in the room, really hear it not just re-imagine it. I stared at myself in the motel mirror and thought I looked odd, driven crazy by her instigating the ending. Should I do it? Suicide? No, I've a son.

I studied the flyer advertising my reading tour and the face didn't look anything like me. It was someone else, an imposter on the poster. I lay wide awake all night long and couldn't understand anything about anything.

I was to read at Bright next morning and got up out of bed like a woozy Lazarus at about six and drank black coffee and plenty of sugars and obediently sipped my Nutri-Grain with canned diabetes tropical fruit in it with tons of fresh cold milk for energy.

The mobile book truckdriver banged on my door at 7 am exactly and drove fast to Bright, which was just as vivid as its name, with magnificent scribbly, gnarled gum trees and fantastic hills and sheep chatting to one another everywhere and magpies carolling with harelips, and we chatted away merrily enough and pulled into Bright nice and punctual. She introduced me to the Bright Library staff and I was escorted into a really cosy big function room all set up nice and gay with fresh flowers picked for me set in crystal vases. They all knew me from the *Sun News*

Pictorial articles I'd written twenty-five years before; they could recite from them.

I said a few things they liked and they even clapped some remarks I made up on the spot, and they asked me how my family was and that was pretty hard to answer when it's over. I spoke good-naturedly and friendly, as I am mostly that way, but my mind left me way behind and it sped away on its chaotic own, delivering unto me hundreds of disastrous images to wreck the reading; it was like sixteen forms of schizophrenia.

I was fighting my selves, as it were, and they were at war. The ancient ladies continued to clap and smile as though to say 'Barry is our own dear boy!' They clucked and kissed me and asked for my autograph and said they'd bought my latest book, which could easily have been twenty years ago, and said, 'Could you make that out to Jill in hospital? She hasn't got long to go and has always loved you in print, dear boy of the ordinary battlers.' I just about fell over.

We drove back to Wangaratta after the Bright ladies had put on an old-fashioned scone and tea celebration and I shook hands with boring and exciting people at the same moment, not having a clue what was going on in any way. I had brain damage.

My chauffeur seemed in a perfect froth all the way back through the heavenly landscape, for all she spoke of was what pricks men were and how they were all control freaks and how they didn't deserve to be born and she was giving me an earache. The diesel fumes in the suffocating vehicle gave me vertigo and a sharp headache too. I got back to the idiotic motel and collapsed.

The phone rang and it was the next library, Myrtleford, reminding me not to be late nor to be overserious with the members of their library as some of them had cancer. I said that would be okay and swallowed a fistful of Stilnox sleeping capsules that didn't work for a second; all I did was mime resting. The motel bed was my lumpy assassin. No wonder my wife had had enough of me. The anxiety was getting worse. It was just awful and went on from the time I woke to the time I conked. Misunderstanding what people say. Misunderstanding what I'm to say.

Not long ago I was teaching cartooning and verse at Benalla West Primary School and the kids liked me. We drew all kinds of amusing things, such as comical poodles with bouffant hair extensions. I was okay a month ago, wasn't I? I had always gone out to people and loved strangers rather than feared them but now I could feel anxious at a laidback gathering like a child's happy birthday party.

Suddenly everything has a million angles and nothing is simple.

One's wife has left one.

I had to cancel the rest of the tour I got so sick, like some sort of perversity or mania. Had it always been in me or just the last month and getting much more advanced? Self-conscious and deluded and not listening but interrupting. Some of my best friends are in Benalla but I had to cancel and drove home like a man without conscience or memory. I hated myself. I needed professional help. She had to instigate that.

I suppose I was okay to drive on the highway; I have always liked motoring. I got home to our Carlton terrace and could give no account of the tour to my wife and son. We ate our curry and rice and I read to my sweet son in his doubledecker bed in the normal sort of fatherly way, and he went to sleep on my shoulder in the normal sort of way, but my mind was accelerating and racing off a precipice.

In the morning I was supposed to appear as poet in residence at Camberwell Grammar School for a week of teaching middle school, but I stayed in bed and did absolutely nothing, I didn't even ring them or feel tragic or ashamed about not turning up, which honestly isn't like me, really it isn't. It was the depression. It flattened me. I had zero guilt. No conscience.

After a week of this kind of errant behaviour my wife took me for tests at the local St Vincent's Hospital where the specialists could see just how ill I was, partly because I couldn't make any sort of sense and partly because it was obviously a crisis. I got a referral to the clinic, the perfect spot for disappearing cognitive powers, the power to speak and think. Would they return my family and my humour to me?

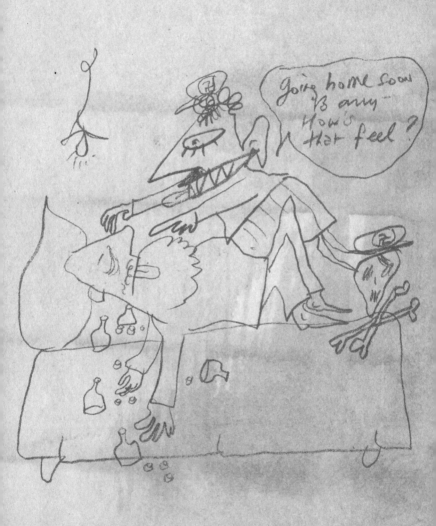

Chapter
three

THE CLINIC WAS supersonic-surgical, as these places mostly are, with oppressive air-conditioning that keeps you too warm or clammy; it needs to be altered but no one will dare change it one degree in temperature because it was set at an exact high warmth ten years ago and its long history of perspiring patients have just had to put up with it, feeling too hot that is, all the time, in the corridors and in the interview rooms and in your awful wakeful bed.

I nervously completed the admission forms and terms of conditions paperwork and did a great deal of gulping in disbelief as my wife accompanied me into Room 5, which would be my new home for sixty nights in a row, a long time to recover; I thought it would be only a few days. My wife packed my neat clothes in wardrobes and sets of drawers and there was nothing more to say really, although we are separate we are still friendly, kind of.

'Look after yourself and I'll bring Louis in tomorrow after work, he's dying to see you.' She's gone.

A huge, well-built Malaysian-looking lady called Sharna fussed around me and insisted on me having a shower but I didn't really want one so it turned into a violent argument with her raising her voice at me and screaming out that I shouldn't disappoint my son by smelling. 'You do in fact smell,' she yodelled and handed me a big block of cacky soap and pointed to the shower in a no-mucking-around kind of a way.

'I don't need one,' I explained and she looked like she was going to strike me in the face. She's a pugilist. She's my enemy – soap!

'You want to be able to be relied upon when you go back to your job, don't you?' she said, foaming away at me, coming up close to me and shoving the soap into my chest then handing me a towel. She was not going to back down and imperiously demanded I take a shower immediately if I wanted to recover from depression, which is closely related to taking a shower, she pointed out, with bared teeth that were vile and yellowish. She looked like a sheepdog with those fangs.

'I can't take a shower with you in the room,' I replied, but she refused to budge and defiantly folded her muscular arms and grated her teeth and just waited me out, so in a bad temper for being bested I dropped my pants and held the pot stomach in and shivered involuntarily and in a marked fashion turned on the hot water.

She was still out there. I could sense her presence from the shower that bit into my back, bringing no relief only unwanted heat on my skin. Truth is, I hadn't washed properly for ages and was filthy in the extreme, and I knew she was right but I was not used to being upstaged and hated her in my unreasonable way. Everything about me was so unreasonable and questioning and awkward and miserable.

I had to get dressed in front of her, a perfect stranger, and it was embarrassing but she wouldn't lose out; she was absolutely determined on it, and looked so furiously into me. 'That feels better, doesn't it?'

'No!'

She vipered at me like no one ever has before, not even my worst enemy. 'You must learn to respect yourself if you want to recover!' she shouted; she actually shouted at me, less than one inch from my face. 'You have been lying in your bed doing nothing but damage to yourself, have you no pride? You have a tremendous responsibility and that responsibility is to be capable of taking proper care of your thirteen-year-old son you claim you adore so much. If you want to return to the living you must do simple deeds such as willingly washing your bloody body!'

I sighed and did up my belt and put on my slippers without the socks inside them as the odd socks were all wet and crumpled up and dripping, so she personally knelt before me and put on my white socks herself. She tugged them up so tightly and made sure they matched, in her short-sighted opinion, before she also put my slippers on properly; she'd been in my room for a full thirty minutes, easily, and I wonder how she knew how much I adore my son, but possibly I told her as soon as we met but I can't remember anything anymore, that's the thing of it. Nothing.

She was so crude and such a complete peasant, I thought in my arrogant confusion, but she was simply trying to teach me the most important lesson in all life, and that is to be able to take care of your body. That before the damaged brain. First things first. She was right.

'Your shirt is filthy!' she hissed and shoved it in the washing machine not far away. This was within the first hour of being there as their patient or was it that I've no sense of time? I realised I hadn't washed properly for a long time and didn't shampoo the outer self. It is always more important to write than bathe, as far as I'm concerned, even though I'm forever pressuring my son to hop in the bath.

I got to bed and explained that I was exhausted but she jerked me out of the sheets and one top blanket by the arm and refused to allow me to go into gloom in the early morning bed, to just lie there blank and tapping my feet like pistons due to a forced restlessness and loneliness that can be cured by a simple action like washing.

My first day in the Unit began with what you might call washing-bullying. The rage that is her face was palpable; I could see up close and personal tiny veins pulsing away in her bubbly tannish forehead. 'If you don't want to remain a vegetable, which is what your job is at present, lying of no use in bed and distressing your hard-working wife and making your sweet son fret with anguish about your decision not to live, you *will* wash your body in front of me!' In a rage I disrobed and savagely kicked my pants onto the shower floor. 'Not in that careless fashion, they will get wet that way, sopping wet!' She plucked up the pants and quickly folded them up on the bed and handed me a block of soap and a big bottle of shampoo and pointed to the shower. 'Get in!' she just about foamed at the lips.

I took off my putrescent favourite shirt, the dark blue one, ripping several buttons off in the process and they reverberated on the white ceramic tiles; she bent in agony and picked them all up painstakingly and cupped them in her calloused brown hand. I was so vague I turned on only the hot and scalded myself and then fiddled round with the cold and in the end made a dreadful mess. I had to accept I had met my match and almost smiled. She conquered me just then. Her crisp uniform and starched stockings and stiff hair and imperious Madame Tussaud expression was too much for my pigheadedness.

I was fully dressed now and seated properly on the bed but she grabbed a hair dryer and powerzoomed through my straggly unkempt beard and unbrushed locks. With one arm just about strangling me, she bent over me and dried me down. 'One day you will be of use!' I stared at my own shoes and had no idea who this lady was or where I was. 'You are very sick, you are a very sick person!' She was right.

Everything in me wanted to retreat, burrow, hide in the bed again, escape her. She held me by the right hand and forced me to the lift and she pushed the button and took me into the dining room on the ground floor, where a whole lot of withdrawn people were picking at cutlets and piles of mashed pumpkin. Some depressed patients were only children who nibbled halfheartedly at the food or went out in the butt garden and inhaled their crates of cheap cigarettes.

There was a large cartoon mural of the clinic on the canteen wall that depicted recovering patients and pelicans swishing around and comical speech bubbles all to do with becoming better and going home again. Sharna piled up a huge plateful of hideous hot mashed muck and string beans and peas and greasy crumbed cutlets; she handed me tools to eat them with and demanded instant consumption. She may as well have been holding spanners and hammers. Her eyes were blazing with hate. 'If you don't want to deteriorate, you will eat all what you now see here!' I don't want it, I told her and she ground her back teeth down to the stumps, saw her chance and moved in on me. Because I was sick and knew it, I just sat and tried meekly to outstare Sharna but she was too grinding and tough and had patched up lots of lost fathers.

The other patients coughed and spooned and forked and gulped and fidgeted at their food as I put my mucky plate in the section for mucky plates, and I noticed how rough the sick people were as they cast their remains of food all over the place; then the noble, poorly paid cleaners were soon onto it and whisked the filthy stacks of plates and gluggy spoons and coagulated knives away in a second without a fuss.

It was about noon and I crossed to the lift and observed how a bell tingled in a 'ping!' way every time it jerked to an abrupt halt and every time it 'pinged' everyone turned round hoping that meant there'd be a visitor, but mostly it was just 'pinging', electronic loneliness.

Sharna looked cross as two sticks as I whirled around to see her at the lift. She was very angry and colossally disappointed with me, an old, brain-damaged father. I lay defiantly in the bed and recalled the recent MRI scan at the Epworth Hospital; God, I was so frightened and held the guy's hand as they put me into the big vault-thing to see how damaged my brain was. I had drunk since I was twenty or thereabouts so it was decades of damage. All the deceased drinking companions still calling out to me from the tombstone. Pubs were my companions and ice and whiskey conquered the boredom. Smoking and boozing every conceivable poison in every city in Australia. Drinking backstage, drinking with my wife in the giggling courtyard, my little boy coming up the stairs in our terrace laughing at me unconscious on the dusty top floor.

I have drunk two bottles of white wine and stubbies on top and then cooked burnt steak for the family; it was forty degrees and we had no air-conditioning. My wife refused to have it so I was fried. She said air-conditioning destroys the ozone layer. Raving away hysterically, telling the same old stories, some new ones that have exploded out of the fug of alcohol, I got up the stairs at just seven at night.

'Daddy, it is too bright in the sky to go to sleep, it's far too bright in the sky for it, Daddy!' He burst into bright sarcastic infantile chuckling and tried to rouse me from my blackout and I did wake up for a second and squinted at the angel. He looked a perfect mixture of beauty and disappointment. It was his disappointment that eventually stopped me drinking. I stopped the intake. It was easy.

There is nowhere to go but divorce.

My disappointed, tired-out wife was watching *Seinfeld* on Channel Ten with her aching teacher's feet up on the end of the sofa. I tried to suck up to her by pouring her a wine but she held up her palm in protest so I hit the courtyard again to drink more out there. But I didn't. It's easy to hit the cork back in. My son comes first.

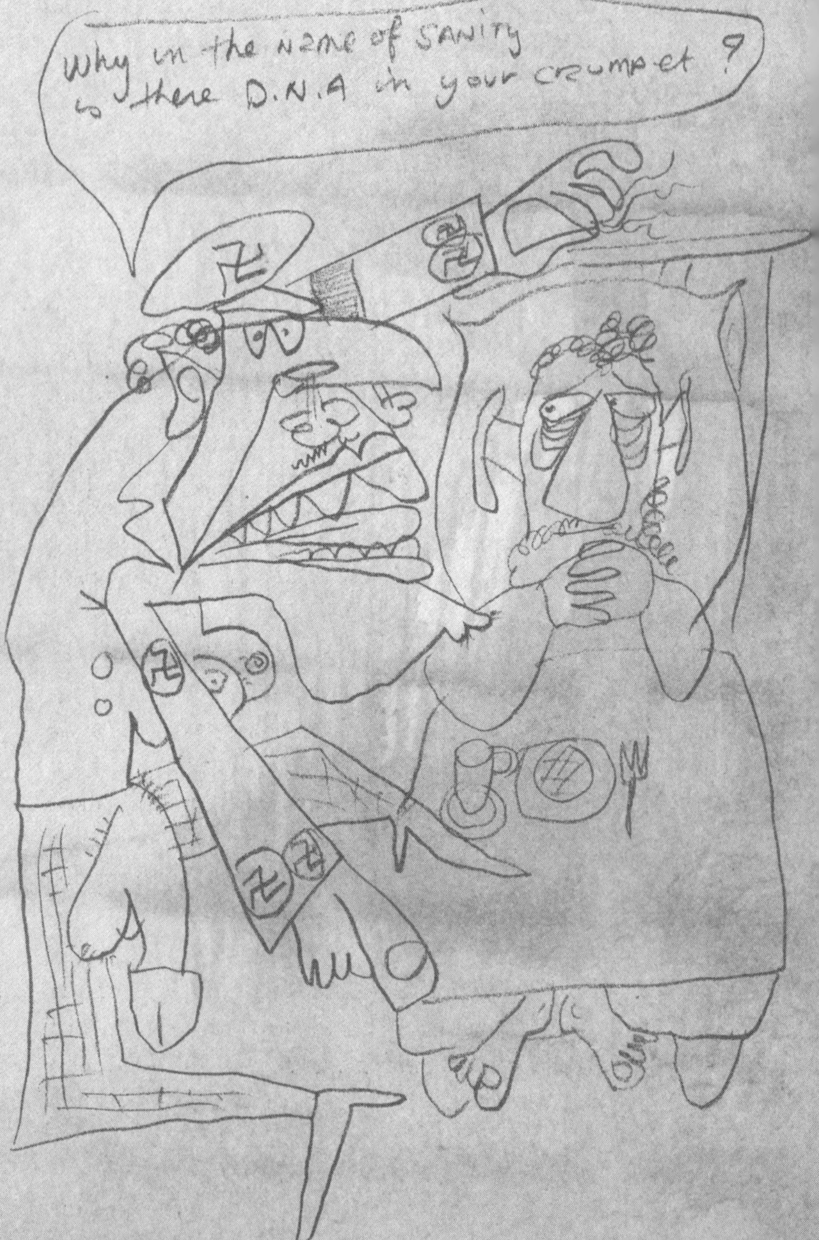
why in the name of sanity is there D.N.A in your crumpet ?

Chapter
four

Now it was two in the afternoon in the Unit. The nurses kept entering Room 5 where it was like a sauna and chastised me for being indolent but I felt close to death and wanted to curl up and cark it. A nurse named Rhonda came in and smiled benignly as she knelt by the bed and stuck a Post-It fluorescent yellow square piece of paper on the chest of drawers with my jocks in it. I put my two-buck glasses on and studied the pencil hieroglyphic. DOCTOR GILBERTSON WILL SEE YOU AT 8 AM TOMORROW MORNING IN INTERVIEW ROOM 2. Why didn't she just tell me.

He was my psychiatrist apparently and was the epitome of haste. Polished bald pate and heroically built and brisk and cocksure and revered by all the staff. He ran rather than walked quickly. He also declined to take the pinging lift as he was a fitness freak and leapt like a bat up the stairs clutching his strange black fold-up briefcase-trolley-notebook-thing.

I hated him.

But he was determined to fix me, do me up, recall me to life.

The evening before I met him I dawdled in the canteen, sort of eating whatever it was all the others were poking at. I met a bipolar man named Kevin who is up and down like the elevator filled with conspiracy theories but droll and enjoyable and huge; he paces round restlessly continually, eating his depression away in towering platefuls.

At eight it's 'Meds' time, which means drug time, and the inmates gather round the dispensary for big night hits. A little paper beaker of water and rinsed-down magic tablets that have the remarkable power to dispense with suicidal thoughts, disastrous images in the head's cinema, feelings of no-worth, memories of being interfered with by a parent. One gulps as one is bid. Many gulps in fact. There's both a feeling of excitement and a guarantee of oblivion.

Their Christian names are cheerfully called out and one after the other they spiral up for their cures, some obsequious, others gruff, some sourly and others like the lost children they really are, unwanted as cancer; it is the outsideness that gets to you the most, they are completely outside everything. They appear to have abandoned their right to live. They support grief. They love to weep. They never sleep or rest without drugs. One young woman swallowing heaps of drugs has a baby but not here, at home with her husband who brings it in every night for her to see but not hold as she is afraid due to her mental condition; the husband is quite positive about it all, boisterous even. But she doesn't want to live and her psychiatrist slowly adjusts her dosage till it's massive. She chainsmokes in the fuggy courtyard and chats hysterically all the time to the chainsmoking others there. This was day one and already it felt like a hundred years of sadness.

An obese Greek lady named Sylvia was the unhappiest face I'd ever seen. She complained incessantly about the food and the uncomfortable bed, and walked round in a sort of rolling disapproval of everything, her roly-poly arms swinging as she circumnavigated her compatriots, watching anything in the common room, the Panasonic television on too loud. They cackled at the advertisements.

We were later dished up squishy fat wholemeal sandwiches on impressive platters. The staff never tired of serving us all sorts of unwieldy food, such as massive wet sandwiches the patients rammed down their gobs as they stared in an unseeing way at the Bob Jane T-Mart television advertisements as though they were a movie.

I got myself photographed at some time that day, first day, and when I got my sedatives just before, I couldn't make myself out in the computerised blow-up of me stuck onto my blue drug basket with sticky tape. There was white medication powder all over my cracked lips as if I was a drooling imbecile.

Sylvia very loudly moaned about not being visited but perhaps her family were too depressed to come in?

Maybe I became so compliant and went along with everything they wanted me to do but they seemed to pamper the patients too much, particularly with the incessant servings of chocolate sponge and sliced watermelon the patients gutsed into, its pink juice going right down their front all the time; not many bothered with finesse or paper serviettes or the usual table manners, so that food went everywhere and the staff were forever cleaning up after them. It was a piggery.

I went to bed that first evening dry-mouthed, drugged to the hilt and as dazed as a shock-victim. The ward was boiling hot and I got up restless and haggard, finding it an absolute swelter in Room 5. I needed to scream but was too conservative to do it.

The aluminium windows were so sealed you couldn't possibly open any of them. The big door to my tomb was painted an awful olive. The vinyl carpet had plastic fibres sailing out of it that stuck in your eyeballs. My clothes looked familiar and unfamiliar as though they weren't part and were part of my past. I wanted to walk in the street and get out but felt meek without strength or courage.

After midnight and still the nurses paced about and their Christian names were announced upon the PA system, as there was a George Orwell microphone at the front desk on level three, where we were, which they just loved to use.

'Rhonda to the front desk, please; Rhonda!'

'Tim to the front desk, please; Tim!'

'Jill to the front desk, please; Jill!'

We'd all been sedated but now we're awakened.

Doesn't this make everyone much more depressed, much more anxious? Why do they make all these inane announcements?

Why not just go and get them; they're only two feet away.

But that is the bureaucracy and you just have to take it.

I tried lying perfectly still in the impenetrable bed but I couldn't discover any peace. The drugs wouldn't kick in. It's five hours since I've swallowed them. The door opened and it's Tim the large London-born nurse and he plonked himself down on the end of my horrid bed. He looked straight into me like a masculine telescope. I regarded him like a snake. 'How you feeling at this stage of the game?' It's 2 am, for God's sake. I actually couldn't get myself to reply as I really felt like topping myself.

'Not bad, Tim,' was all I could manage at this stage of the mental game.

'You look a tad down.'

I didn't feel it. I felt like going to sleep but the tablets didn't do it.

'Well, that is because your system isn't used to them.'

He told me not to sleep with my pants on then left as though he never came. The big, olive, thickish door banged loudly and I heard his big sandals muffle down the hallway. Flippity-floppity-flip.

'Tim to the front desk, please; Tim!' He was actually already there, but it was the official adoration of announcements that turned the staff on.

I actually slept but restlessly so until 6 am when the announcements of Christian names started up again, and it seemed more insistent this time, with more names than ever called.

'Jill to the front desk, please; Jill!'

'Rhonda to the front desk, please; Rhonda!'

Giant bipolar Kevin was gorging up herculean bowls of All-Bran and shimmering litres of skim milk and gooey prunes and he was raving away to both himself and Dee, who has a profound fear of crowds, who went to Brunswick Street the other day on leave, she got leave, and became frightened of her old friends in the trendy latte bars and biscuit bars and had to grab a taxi back to the Unit.

Big tragic Kevin pulled apart many miniature All-Bran cartons and the empty packets lay scattered all over his table. He was remarkably intelligent and awfully scared, of what he could not say, perhaps everything. Me included. He had hate and love in his bulbous eyes. I sort of liked him, but never really trusted him.

Children on narcotics were admitted today at noon and they looked like they still had baby fat on them. They wore dreadlocks and facial jewellery and their minds jumped like rabbits.

I actually tended to trip right over them as I couldn't see where they were because they just propped anywhere they liked and conferred with each other in a conspiratorial kind of way; or a paranoid kind of way, a martyred kind of way. Their parents came in and looked worse than they did. More down. That's the word you heard all the time in the corridors. Down.

The regal way names were called out was at counterpoint

to relaxation classes that were also announced in a very loud and impromptu manner; you never knew when another fascist relaxation class would come up; they were perennial as the notion of suicide. The relaxation classes were tense, very tense.

I went to one of them after a fortnight and just sat in it crosslegged; that was about all I could manage, being a bit of a tub. I tried to pull the gut in but it has a will of its flabby own and all I could do was breathe hard. A blonde pushy English bitch ran the relaxation class as though it were an army drill. Some emaciated sick ones got off on it and did precisely what they were told by the Pom with the Jayne Mansfield bust. At least her tits were fit. The depressed perved on them.

Others like me, pushing sixty, went to the canteen and gutsed into cream biscuits. Anything for a bit of sweetness, including obesity. Sharna took me back into my room at three in the afternoon and we quarrelled about my dirtiness again; she won out and I had to scrub-up in front of her as she stood there, arms folded and back jaw locked like a lock-out, like she lived only for this minute of standing over me and forcing me to dig all the grime and sweat out of my worthless hide. That's how I felt after fourteen days. Worthless.

She locked Room 5 and in a very satisfied and smug sort of way she retrieved from a pocket of her dress a wand rather like a remote television control object and as I stared she pointed it at my unmade bed and the unmade bed that never afforded me rest rose in the air until it was levitated seven feet off the carpet and came to computerised rest well above my head. Now what?

She contrived to make the idiotic bed go up and down many times in a quick way. Then when I was quite giddy at its ups and fast downs she made it, with a perfect hospital tuck in a standout way, like the way she did hospital tucks would win a world prize or something special like that. Then she folded the pink quilt made of nylon and tucked that on top of the laser-tucked bedsheets. She then glared hard into me and read the riot act.

'To recover from your illness you must learn to tuck your sheets in properly and now you have a bed-mobile you may raise your bed upward to seven feet and make sure from underneath that it is done right. Here is your bed-mobile now. Put it somewhere you won't forget, like in your bedside drawer or in the wardrobe under a book you are reading.' She then left and I lay on the bed a foot higher than usual.

It was Angela who saved me. She I liked much more than any of the others there, can't say why; it had to do with an inner beauty like my son's inner beauty. An unassailable love of life you can't purchase. She bossed me around and reminded me to never be lazy or I'd lose the respect of my thirteen-year-old boy and that's right, Angela, you're right, I would. 'You have to get up at six and go to the toilet and do wee then wash your body and put all your clothes on your body and put on clean socks and highly polished neat shoes then rinse your dentures and check your mail and pay any outstanding domestic accounts and then penetrate your porridge and prunes for energy then have a quick peruse of the paper then run for the morning train to work.' That was poetry to me.

'What if I have no work, Angela?'

'That doesn't even come into it, Mr Dickins. You simply have to be ready even if you have no work. Because you never know when things may change in your life and you'll be given work, even if it's not the job you actually want, like digging a ditch or being in the army.' Then she adhered a bright, square, blindingly bright fluorescent Post-It note on my bedside bureau that had DOCTOR GILBERTSON WILL SEE YOU AT NOON TODAY IN INTERVIEW ROOM 2. I couldn't wait.

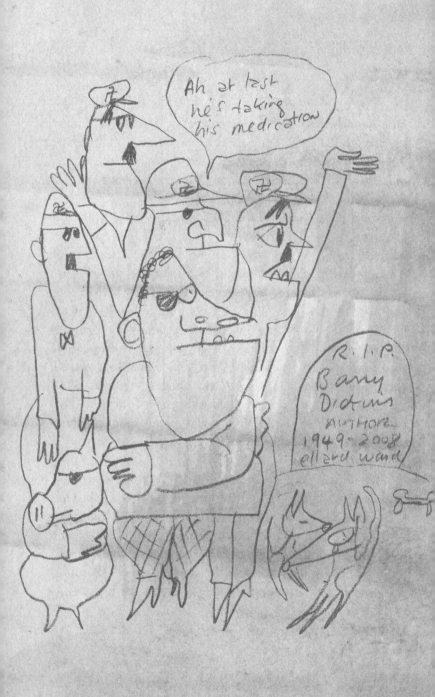

Chapter
five

HE WALKED IN HIS hydraulic way past the front desk and briskly conversed with Angela. Everything he does is brisk, even talking quickly as if talking slowly is sick instead of the reflective, enjoyable conversation I am used to. His black suit is fit for my funeral and black big shoes skid over his invisible shadow. He takes telephone calls quickly and thinks quickly and answers quickly and keeps saying I'm deteriorating.

I tell him I thought I looked up this morning after so many antidepressants last night and then he asks me to tell him their names, or is my memory so bad I can't, even if they went into my system only last night at the medication window where we all hang out for them. Why is he so aggressive? He has a confrontational style and not the bedside manner I'd hoped for. Of course I can't remember the drugs' names even though I've been on them two weeks; one of them knocks me off to sleep and all the others fight the anxiety that screws me up more than anything else, the increasing anxiousness that bites into my head and demands more negative energy be given to it in the name of anguish. The anxiety is worse than the depression by far.

'Surely you can recall their names, you only had them last night, don't you care about what you take? See whether you can

39

remember just one of their names. What day is it today? Where are you? You have no idea of the day, have you? Is it Monday or not? Not Monday? Why is it you don't sleep properly? You keep on talking about your wife wanting a separation but why does she want one? Why have you drunk so much all your life? Why are you fidgeting and trembling? We'll increase your medication I think.'

I now need to fidget. I feel all dry in the throat and it really hurts me to swallow. My eyes sting in a lethal fashion and my shoulders ache as though I've slept on pure concrete. It is the terrible tension of the marriage break-up that's making me ache all over. I don't want the marriage over but she does, so it is, it really is. We once had loads of fun. Twenty-nine years of it.

'One of the nurses on night-duty says you do strange things at night such as wander round carrying linen all evening; I mean, why would you want to do something like that? Apparently you stack bed quilts up in a big mountain in your room, don't you? Why?'

He's right, I do. Last night I went drugged to a large cupboard containing all the linen for the third floor and for some reason I piled it all up high around me, fifteen quilts, thickish quilts and I suppose I did it to give the room some character. I don't know why. To make my room human.

'Why would you do a thing like that?' He neither smiles nor frowns but somewhere judgemental in between. I wish he would chew or something; he is so chaste and immobilised. In Interview Room 2 he is in his element. Entering every single thing I say by pen in a great exercise book that eventually blossoms into my life story. I tell him I think the reason I moved all the bed quilts around was to lend my room some character. He just continues to stare at me.

The tinnitus in my head is vibrantly louder suddenly, almost unbearable. I want to cry out. The more he inquires of me the louder my head is until I need to get up off the black vinyl chair and head for some sort of garden to avoid the two-bit analysis.

'Do you know the date of today? What clinic are you in? Do you think you are deteriorating? There's no doubt that you're deteriorating.'

A week went by in a deteriorating way and I tried to sleep in to catch up but Angela and Sharna were like sheep dogs nipping at my heels, nagging and reminding and repairing and being put out and waking me if I didn't come to heel as my life happened to be on the line. They were bringing me back – recalling me to life.

The Beijing Olympics were on the giant television and it seemed a bit ironic: the blurry patients chomped on the triangular-cut wedges of watermelon and generous slices of chocolate sponge watching Korean ping-pong champions belting the tiny white celluloid ball at over 140 kph. The lethargy and the archery. The stupefaction and the hurdling. The chomping and the weightlifting. The isolation and the hundred metre dash.

It was late at night and still they trotted out the food. Trays of cake and bulgy tomato sandwiches with lashings of thick white pepper so some of them sneezed as they viewed the high diving and sighed as the sleek athletes completed a quadruple pirouette into the televised blue chlorine, hardly making a splash as the tireless nurses fetched more chronic indigestion. The hospital farted all night loudly.

A perennially cheerful man called Ian, who joyously helped out with the ECTs down in the Recovery Room, was plonking down various cut-up fruit salads and winking at patients and saying, 'How's it going, Kevin' and 'How's it going, Sally' constantly but Kevin and Sally were quite without life and didn't bother to answer Ian. The breathtaking feats of fitness continued apace as the patients ate without energy or enthusiasm, more like the plump sandwiches were actually eating them.

She wants to leave me so I shall live with my son in a motel. Make his lunch on the miniature bench underneath the overhead telly. I told her I still adore her but she just lights another smoke and puffs it looking down. Right in my eyes she repeats that she doesn't feel anything for me. But she comes into the hospital to visit me after a hard day of teaching school and all that driving in peak traffic, driving our son to school at eight in the morning and teaching class all day and ordering a renovation for our terrace in Carlton.

How did I lose her? I can't remember what we quarrelled about and she can't remember either.

Now that's a funny thing. Here I am getting shock-therapy to cheer myself up and she tells me during her visit she doesn't feel love for me anymore, just friendship, but what's that? It's great to see her tuck into the food in the canteen when she comes in. She and Louis enjoy their salads and juicy pieces of roast chook and glass of fruit juice and in a way it is like home. I know each particular eating habit and mannerism of teaspoon and fork and the way they chew and nibble and swallow is all in the script of love. We gossip and giggle like normal and her leaving me seems perfectly absurd, but she's doing it all right, after years, she assures me, of not feeling anything. One night in the canteen she said in a depressed, downcast kind of way, picking at her rice with her plastic fork, 'Maybe we could give it another go.' But that just demoralised me even more the way she said it in the gloomy canteen. You can't feign love or pretend affection but why now when I'm in a psychiatric hospital?

I kept on remembering meeting her when she first interviewed me twenty-seven years ago. When we first started going out is still current in my functioning memory machine, my mind still works okay. The baby coming through in 1995. How sick she was at his birth; she could easily have died of the incredible complications. Thank God she did not. She won't hold me and won't touch me but she will visit me.

My little boy jumps on my back when he comes in.

We 'verse' each other at table tennis in the Recreation Room and scream out and chortle. He is uncanny with any form of ball and I have played tennis and footy with him ever since Sarah gave him birth. He loves to play and is pretty much always happy; in fact his cheeks puff up when he's joyous and the laughter he produces manufactures joy in me as soon as I hear it start up because the depression goes.

Sarah laughs too, the way we play ping-pong and bound around after the balls making plenty of racket. She has ordered a hip replacement for Christmas and is in agony with it in July. She is not my enemy but a ghost now of dead love and worthless affection.

I accompanied both to the lift and of course it 'pings' loudly as it always does when the patients' necks whirl round and they expect a visitor. She limps with the pain she is experiencing and loses the car keys as she always does, then I watch her start up her stationwagon and depart in blue fumes of goodbye. When I waved farewell as she drove off it felt good as well as terrible. She left freshly ironed pants.

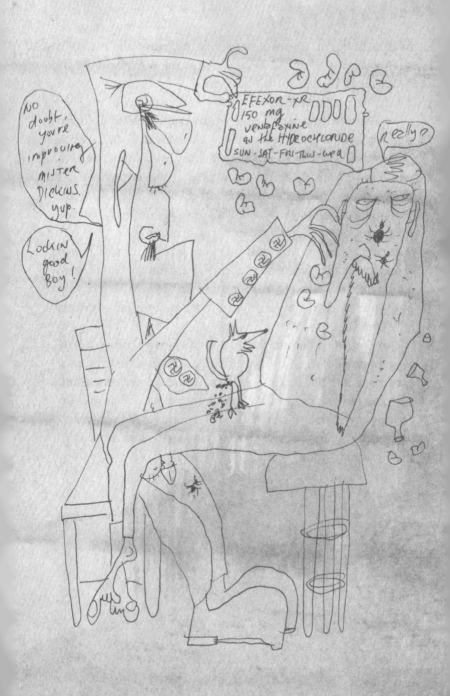

Chapter
six

To GO BACK TO THE blank bed, to not be able to write was unreal to a writer like me, who writes each day or just about: articles for the newspapers and stage plays and poems to read on the radio or the television or live. I depressed back to Room 5 and discovered a brand-new Post-It note on my bedside table, adhered there by nice Rhonda who was always buoyant and naturally easygoing and telling me I can get back, that I can do it, and she really liked my wife and son Louis. DOCTOR GILBERTSON WILL SEE YOU AT NINE TOMORROW MORNING IN INTERVIEW ROOM I. Funny how he wanted 1 instead of 2. It had always been 2 all along where we couldn't communicate.

Sitting with the others outside the medication dispensary, I felt filleted. Like my heart and soul had been slid out. Like I'd never teach again or draw with children or do anything creative again after thirty-six years of comedies and dramas and appearing on telly on all the channels as a raconteur, joking without scripts.

There is definitely a positive eagerness to the way the nurses dispense the medication here, a joy to see the patients float through a sea of costly addictive pharmaceuticals. Ian administers the drugs with such unabated glee he positively glows with inner contentment and fascination for mood-swings. Here are the astonishingly active tablets that kill those annoying mood-swings. Leaving the recipient with nothing in the noggin. Your head is like a scooped-out canteloupe.

I just beheld Ian in the Recovery Room helping with the ECT, now here he is giving out hundreds of anti-trauma capsules, anti-anxiety drops. It's a candy-fest. The patients look so drab hanging out for their tablets and sort of talk with each other but sort of don't at the same time because they are so destroyed by their own lives. They know they are dead people. Like me.

Why have they got me on Seroquel? More American poison: 25 mg of anti-psychotic nonsense. The psychiatrist informs me the Seroquel are to make me sleep. I looked them up in some drug dictionary and they're for schizophrenia, which luckily I don't get.

Great big atomic nurses and tiny automatic ones, it doesn't matter. They all help. Sickness is such a hindrance. I've always been well over the span of my nearly six decades. I had my teeth out at twenty; that's pretty normal for a poet. I had ten days at Ballarat Base Hospital in 1999 due to chronic food poisoning that resulted in septicaemia and that was pretty serious, I suppose.

My enormous, long white-bearded supervisor at Ballarat University Drama Department, Bruce Widdop, bought me a family pizza to celebrate opening night of a student season of monologues, and unbeknownst to me it contained human shit. I ate half without of course knowing that, and nearly came to my death due to all the poisons inside me. A junkie cook had made the salad without washing his hands after going to the loo to wipe his bottom. That's probably the worst thing that ever happened to me, I suppose.

Now my days are ironed out with so many meetings with my psychiatrist choreographed via Post-Its.

'Do you know what day it is?'

No.

'Do you know where you are?'

The Unit.

'That's very good.'

Jesus, is it?

He is completely crouched like a metallic coil over his exercise books, duly writing in it every single thing I tell him. Why doesn't he shout himself a tape recorder? It's all done with a black biro, the whole saga.

'I'm going to increase your antidepressants.'

But I already feel dopey every morning, so out of it I don't know what I'm doing.

'It's to lift your mood and complement your ECT, which I'm going to increase as well.'

I don't know if I want ECT anymore. I feel just awful after it.

'Do you want to slide back?'

I'm not going to slide back. I want to live.

'You have a long history of sliding back. Look at your disastrous cancelled Wangaratta author's tour in March, for example.'

What's that got to do with it?

'All you did after the tour was lie in your bed while your wife went to work teaching.'

You're trying to make me guilty.

'But that is a fact, isn't it? Your wife goes to work while you go to bed?'

All through April I was deluded and out of my mind, that's right, it came to me in April the terrible thing and devoured my conscience wholesale. I remember going back to bed – not tired – and staying there one whole Saturday when my little boy had a tennis match on out in Watsonia, a long way from innercity Carlton; he had to be there by eight in the morning and my insomniac wife drove him there. God, was I sick then. Out of my mind.

She had worked a ten- or eleven-hour day doing her teaching and then prepared our supper, out in the kitchen grating carrots and peeling brown onions and chopping up mince and boiling up pasta while I sat on my bottom in our courtyard and chainsmoked and threw down the wine; she came out and joined me from time to time and we joked about the day, and she cautioned me about over-indulging.

I ate my meal drunk and conversed with my son drunk and tried to understand *Seinfeld* drunk, it is understandable drunk, then gone upstairs and looked at my confused face drunk and washed it drunk and went to bed drunk and slept drunk. I kidded myself it was the vile tinnitus that kept me from repose but I drank because I felt like it. Every night I was at the bottle shop buying wine and more smokes and energy drinks for Louis. Not every night but it felt that way. I actually prefer being sober and straight.

Now here I am in rehab sober. Looking at the gifted Sally's patiently painted copies of Vincent Van Gogh's irises. Sally has depression and anxiety like me and she kneels all day in her room on the hard vinyl carpet and mixes up oil colours on little scraps of paper and painstakingly reinterprets Van Gogh's famous pictures to make them her own; it's like she's built her own little art gallery in her inert room. They are all along the wall, maybe twenty altogether, they really are very beautiful and I encourage her to exhibit her pictures, to hold an exhibition somewhere; the afternoon dust motes sail through the sunshine and pick out the highlights of each work of art. It is like she can't credit a drop of praise and looks down at her shoes but I really mean what I say.

'Thanks for your kind compliments, you don't have to do that, I don't expect it.' She mixes up crimson and a dab of white and adds a patient flourish. The identical crimson of her violent blush.

At dinner last night I ate next to an old guy who said he used to be a jazz musician and played professionally at late-night clubs, played the alto sax; he picked at his peas and broad beans and lamb on his dish and confessed he's got cancer of the mouth. We got on really well, but I went to bed feeling so sorry for him.

That lost Saturday when my son played competition tennis an hour-and-a-half drive from our place haunts me as one of the lowest points in my whole life, when some lethal destructive force made me do it, lie there in the upstairs bed and do nothing while she battled through heavy traffic and the rain to get him to tennis comp on time. It is distraction. I didn't care about them or anything of any kind.

Another dreadful time was a Friday morning when for no reason I didn't want Louis to attend school and tried to talk him out of going to a thing he loves. I had trimmed his white bread sandwiches and evenly spread hazelnut topping on them and plonked a nice mandarin and chunk of cake in his red lunch box; we walked for a few sunny streets and the insane part of me, the depressed part said not to bother going to school.

'Whatever for, Daddy?' he said, with a confused expression on his forehead. I told him it was going to rain like mad and that he'd get wet through and I didn't want that to happen to him. It was an anxiety attack. We just stood together in confusion on the footpath near our terrace and he placed his heavy schoolbag down and put his thin arms on his hips in pure exasperation.

'Why do you want to remain indoors all day, Daddy?' he protested. 'Don't you get bored?'

How can I honestly remember why I was like that a few months ago? It doesn't bear scrutiny. It feels unreal like I was never like that.

The psychiatrist informs me that due to alcohol abuse over the years damage has been done to my frontal lobes, not to mention the harm done to my cognitive powers, but I don't think he's correct about any of that stuff. My memory has got me work in the past, it has written the popular columns and the many books, it is the active power of detail in the recollecting that I still do best. It's my best skill. As far as I can recall.

I am still standing there in limbo a few yards from our terrace with my son in his school guernsey and zip-up backpack full of his dutiful homework, science homework, his red plastic lunch box and bathers for school swimming and shoes; he is standing right by me in his white runners looking up at me crushed like a forgotten flower.

But I don't care. I don't care about a thing now it's on me; the anxiety is too strong. He moves from side to side out of summer restlessness because he wants to run, he's a real athlete and here I am still holding him up telling him I don't want him to go to school.

'How can you stand remaining indoors all day, lying on the bed, don't you want to run and hit the ball like we always do?' He is inconsolable and at the point of hot tears of frustration but I don't care.

'Perhaps you're right, Daddy, it is better if I don't go to school today and stay home with you in the house. I'll just watch television or read.'

But then the anxiety lifts and I breathe better and my shoulders relax and I say he is right and really ought to attend school, so he runs across the busy main road but is quite safe – he looked both ways – and I wave goodbye and watch him disappear until I see him again after school. The entire day I lie in bed beyond belief, staring at my haggard old confused face in the bathroom mirror, not eating or sipping, just lying there dispirited and thinking of burial.

These snippets are finicky embroideries of recollections of guilt and fathomless shame from the recent past when I honestly didn't know what I was doing from day to day.

My joyous boy is my raison d'être and we used to play tennis in the park every day, hitting the ball to each other on the path through that jade-green park, doing a thing we used to call a heaven shot, which meant belting the ball so hard upwards it went higher than clouds go, or at least it seemed to, and the fun of it made us both laugh hard. Like my wife, we all lived just for the joy of life.

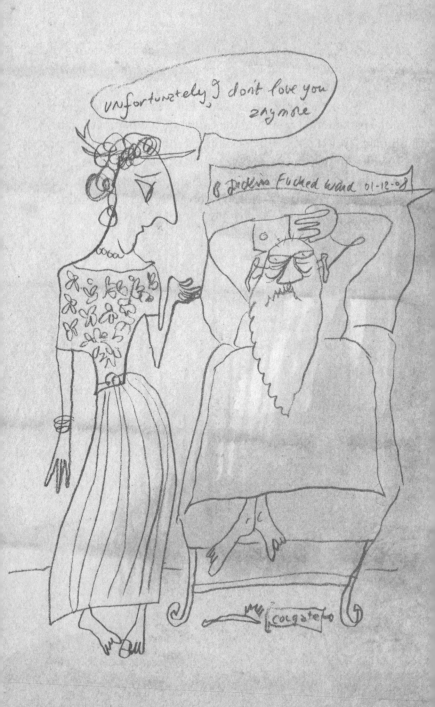

Chapter
seven

TIME SPIRALLING EVER-FORWARD and time travelling ever-back again are the same force in depression. It is well past midnight and I remember the birth of our son, Louis, thirteen years ago at the Royal Women's Hospital in Grattan Street, Carlton. I went into the maternity ward on the third floor with her and she remained in her bed and they handed me a stretcher to lie on. We chatted on long into the birth-night like best friends, for such we were. Are.

In a way it was as though the whole thing was androgynous. Not man nor woman just colleagues on the road through life; companions who have always conversed in an impromptu way like stand-ups. It was as if she wasn't pregnant but just enjoying a rest, albeit a dramatic and agonising one. It was seven at night and all she cared about was the whereabouts of her choice of favourite nighties and her Elizabeth Arden make-up and how much the birth was going to hurt.

She wasn't a very good colour though we still chatted and reminisced about things, like how we met after I came back to Australia in 1982 after living in New York. She'd lived there for years as an au pair for a rich couple; the father beat their son. How long we had fought for the right to bear a baby after years of frustration, it was actually going to happen. A miracle indeed.

The overhead light hurt her eyes a lot and she shielded them from the hurtful rays, and requested lots of water to sip and was getting very uncomfortable by now, the team of nurses scurried around admonishing and reminding and taking her temperature and her face was going black due to dangerous high blood pressure and it is six in the morning and there are no jokes between us now.

I stood patiently by the windows looking out onto familiar Grattan Street, lined with friendly ancient trees containing possums that rushed round precisely like the nurses, though their surface was bark and the frantic nurses' surface was linoleum, and she was sighing and groaning and saying 'Oh, dear!' a great deal, and 'Oh, dear God!' even more.

For some obscure reason the head matron was called Wally Donaldson; I can picture her easygoing countenance as though it were yesterday, a real no-fuss lady of some importance, great importance because I was worrying about Sarah's blood-pressure sailing up so high she could easily die, as afterwards we found out just what a near thing it was.

She is wriggly and excited and happy and eager and puffing and panting, a complete transformation from the shy woman who accompanied me twenty-odd hours back. She grasps the gas hose with feverish determination and pushes the sheath hard over her mouth to get at the gas that is supposed to cut the physical agony, but she says she feels as if she is being carved in half by the coming baby. I'm helpless.

One second I'm gazing abstractly through the ward window at leafy old Grattan Street, a thoroughfare I've walked along all my life as a single bloke, from student to pensioner so to speak, from child to man, disconnected and bachelor again. Free in word and association of sensation, in short a poet of long-standing and a lot of sitting. Now no longer wordsmith or any calling other than friend watching the common miracle of birth. After the first birth there is no other.

The scurrying to increase, the noises to grow greater, the perspiring of the mother to become full-on-sweating and the distress to become terror and the frightened face to become horrified as the baby kicks and the terrible spasms kick her sideways.

'This one coming up is going to sting you,' cautions Wally the relaxed midwife, arms folded. She bends over my wife to inspect the pathway of the sudden baby who shall change everything.

My hysterical wife screams her lungs out and the desperation with which she reaches for and grabs the mask for the gas is more of a lurch, with her fingers uncurled and curling up and hanging onto the gas mask for dear life. She sits bolt upright and is bathed in sweat; she herself calls the sweating revolting and now the nurses crouch in much closer and are all on her. She is screaming and sucking down the gas for all she is worth which is priceless as I have never loved her more than this instant when the baby will come and pluck up our loneliness and what she calls our selfish pleasures. Movies and lunches and all that selfishness.

I am seated right beside her to her left watching intently the exact blood pressure measurement she is experiencing and I don't ever take my eyes off the gauges of the instrumentation depicting her statistics, even though my eyes are really watering from the hot overhead lighting plot, which I wish they'd turn down a notch. This isn't to do with me.

They are rocking her like a baby herself and shushing her and quietening her and desperately trying to relax her but she is quite like a wild animal out of control. Her right fingernails are going straight through my right wrist, all the way through it and hurting me a lot but nothing matters except the baby coming through, and it is, for a nurse holds my head still and gestures to the gap widening where the nut-like top of its head is showing. *His* head. Louis coming.

My wife is hoarsely barking and shrieking in non-English but the old familiar sounds of physical agony and flailing and jerking and eyes lolling and rolling and now staring at me in rage, furious intense wrathfulness that somehow the pain is my fault, and it is, I'm the father after all, now it takes half a dozen of them to keep her flat on the operating bench with its saturated sheets and kicking legs all over the place, so different from all the coy birth books that depict bluebirds and storks and marigolds and so on.

In the midst of all her yelling, Wally the patient midwife gives me, forces me, educates me, elucidates me, guides my fingers to clutch a fuzzy pair of abstract scissors, now she guides my right shoulder and right arm and right hand to snip the umbilical cord which I do through my millions of hot tears. I can hardly see what it is I have to do but Wally who steers me through the common procedure, and now smiles, grins at me as though to say, 'There, it wasn't that hard, was it now?'

The baby is a boy called Louis whom Sarah calls Louis the very second he is delivered alive and plonked in Sarah's strong arms.

'There you are, Louis,' she whispers to him crying his head off in her bosom. 'Where have you been for so long a wait?'

He has always been Louis, long before his real appearance and real eyes and the funny way he never cries, not seldom cries but actually never cries. Not since the birth. A born stoic. He hates fuss: he said that once.

She gets me to go to Myers to buy her a new nightie and new proper slippers, not cheap ones but nice and cosy on the feet; an old nun goes with me on the tram, she just happened to be in the ward where the birth took place, we struck up a nonchalant conversation and she quite made me laugh a few times on the tram, an ecclesiastical raconteur; she escorted me to the right level of Myers where nighties were. She chose the prettiest nightie as well as the slippers with the pompoms on. We chatted as though we were ancient friends, and I bought useless things such as tins of cashews and oddly fragrant Indian soaps and pairs of socks. I purchase without intention.

I lost her somewhere in the crowd and sipped a few coffees and remembered the very first thing my wife said at the point of birth with the newborn baby snug in her muscular arms she smiled at me and said in a soft weak voice, 'Could you be so good as to pop over to that milk bar in Cardigan Street – you know the one – and get me a beautiful fresh cappuccino with lots of sugar in it? Make it three!'

Now it is I who is beginning to feel weary from all the hope and emotion. I carry the goodies in a few Myers carry bags and rush into the Women's Hospital again. My heart she pounds.

For the life of me I cannot recall what lift to get into or what level she's on. I am desperate for a wee because it's been days since I urinated just about. So what I did was run just about into the Gents on the ground floor, but a cleaner has just disinfected it and the slippery white ceramic tiles are awash with wondrous Dettol. There was a big stiff mop in there and everything: a metal bucket and the lid was up.

In the one slapstick pantomime action I performed a cartwheel on the saturated surface and circumnavigated the glistening ceramic white lavatory bowl and ended up striking my mouth with considerable force on the lid and knocked myself out cold. I was unconscious for ten minutes within the toilet still clutching my Myers bags. My lips came up bloated and inflamed and my throat hurt and was all bruised. My suit was soaked and crumpled and rather spoiled.

Like a proper gentleman I gripped the Myers bags and sponged myself down with bits of random dry lavatory paper and caught the elevator to the third level. She had the tiny baby right on her chest and her relaxed hands were so easy with his body. Her eyes were so raccoon-like and all black and dark purple with bloodshot interiors. I looked at the instrumentation of the blood pressure gauges and she was as high as you can get before you die; in fact a nurse informed me it was a near thing.

'You might as well go home and have a sleep and come back tomorrow,' she sighed. I liked her sighs.

'Isn't it miraculous, after so much heartache and never going to term?' She never looked more beautiful or contented and the baby too.

I drove home high on happiness and drank frozen apple juice that had gone off. I fed the cat on Kitekat. I fried some black pudding and gobbled it burnt black on burnt toast with thick sauce on it and lashings of white pepper. Fuel in time of need.

This dozy state is the antithesis of clinical depression. To hit the sack like a happy dead person and pull the blinds down but not in sadness but just to drop out of excitement. I slept in my crumpled suit all day and have never been happier, not once.

In the morning everything was ecstasy, just driving the car in traffic was sheer rapture, the symphonies floating out of the car radio blew my mind, everything did, even the policemen looked angelic. I urinated perfectly this time and never got concussed, not for a single second. She was asleep with the baby asleep when I arrived with the perfect frothy hot takeaway cappuccino. 'You remembered: three sugars. Darling!'

Bouquets kept coming from my employers and her friends; the room was full of fresh-cut flowers that looked like kaleidoscopes.

She was pretty red in the face clutching our newborn baby boy.

The new Myers slippers were still on her bed unwrapped; the mauve tissue had tumbled onto the floor some time ago.

She was in there for three days altogether and then the tiny nuclear family went home together in the family buggy. I made her scrambled eggs on cracked wholemeal thick toast; she was really starving by now, but no coffee as she simply had to sleep, the baby too, of course. The phone rang from *The Age* newspaper wanting a new column so I wrote it straight away. The house was alive again with hope in it and coffee and laughter at anything. This is us at our highest point. Rapt.

You think of these things in a psychiatric institution from time to time, particularly when the psychiatrist they've assigned to your case tells you you're deteriorating.

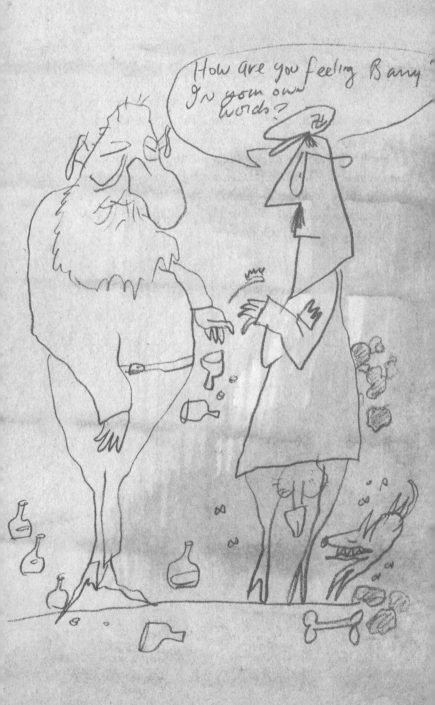

Chapter
eight

It's EIGHT AT NIGHT NOW and the patients are lined up for their medication, me too, and the Ed guy has thrown himself on the carpet in a terrible convulsion and is gripping hard his own clothes, in particular his pants, and is thrashing around in agony sobbing hoarsely and groaning deeply, I ask a fellow patient what's wrong with him exactly and she says he's having flashbacks to some trauma he went through when he was much younger, like being sexually abused by his dad for instance. He seems to be there for some minutes, very long are those fearful minutes of what we used to call epilepsy and madness but it was actually his own father who raped him; now he skids and crashes about and collides with others who simply haven't a clue how to assist him. Two big male nurses carry him back to his room and close his door but those loud sobs can still be heard clear as a bell as we line up for our 'meds', people gossiping and gulping down paper cups full of water and their antidepressants.

'Doctor Gilbertson has put you on new medication,' I am informed at the window. 'Thiamine and Vitamin A to compensate for your years of alcohol.' I throw it all down and do anything they tell me from now on as I am getting restless and dream of getting out.

I try to sleep because I have my second electrocution tomorrow morning and am dreading it absolutely. I have my old white tennis socks on because they are of home. The missing sense of place is getting me down now after six weeks here. Forty-two goddamned days of humiliation and paternalism and loneliness. When one's wife leaves one what exactly can one do? I guess she just found it too hard putting up with my psychosis and mood-swings. But she is very moody herself; or has she forgotten that fault in her own character? She's not so easy to live with either, with all her unpredictable moods such as rage and ill temper that comes from nowhere. Then she's perfectly contented again so soon. We're the same type: manic-depressives.

It is 6.30 am and here they are again, the four of them in my darkened doorway, a reprise of what happened just before. The same sinister silhouettes and the same melancholy lighting like a scene in some opera when the devils come in. A lady holds a big square steel torch aloft without speech, the rays of the stabbing yellow light bite into my sore hay-fevered eyes. They come over.

I am assisted up and put my pants on over my underpants and put my dark blue shirt on and in bare feet accompany the squad of murderers – so they seem – to the pinging lift and soon I see the dead – for they look it – draped over operating-table-looking bed-things, with old arms dangling down and old stern lifeless ghoulish countenances looking at me upside down, having been given ECT they are deceased-looking. Very.

There is a kind of drowsy humour to the shock therapy and in a way nothing could be more natural than seeing patients put out to it; they look precisely like commuters on Melbourne's public transport system after all, all they need is a ticket in their claw. Time to validate.

I am instructed to lie perfectly still and it is done much quicker this time, almost in a perfunctory manner, a taken for granted kind of routine as though I am a shock-therapy veteran after two doses. I watch Ian put the needle in my left wrist so amiably I want to be sick. He is so unctuously unanxious. A greaser. My old heavy head topples onto my left arm as soon as the needle goes in my body. I cry when they hold me flat to put the plastic sheath gas mask on my nose. I feel violated even though they are trying to lift my mood. What's wrong with mood-swings anyway?

Not rushed by quick wheelchairs this time but walked woozy along the infernal halls back to oblivion again, the aroma of lostness to contend with, and no appetite for anything except more tiring unconsciousness, more unwanted drugged repose, sleep this way or that; it isn't fun being so drugged.

The flashback-traumatised Ed guy seems okay now watching the boring Beijing Olympics with all the bored others sucking strength out of watermelon and thick, disgusting white-bread chicken and mayo sandwiches to get through the long night as the high diving heroes perform their predictable somersaults.

Of course it's depressing just being treated for it but the most disagreeable sight here is incredibly wealthy young women being treated for clinical depression and anxiety coupled with post-natal depression; there have to be at least two of these phenomena come in each week, booking themselves in for a cure for suicidal impulses or delusions.

I saw two of them get in the lift just this morning covered with 24-carat jewellery and topaz brooches, with long artificially tanned legs and big busts and oodles of make-up and bizarre thick lips and Italian skirts, pushing high-fashion perambulators containing depressed babies. Their variety of depression seems like the latest trend; their grace and bearing are riveting, and they call each other darling constantly and chainsmoke in the fuggy courtyard, snorting gorgeous nicotine. I've stopped smoking and drinking for the millionth time.

As I consider them I wonder if they have ECT like me.

I tremble something exquisite first thing in the morning, experiencing the new form of convulsive hangover, so different from the years of wine. I haven't been hanging out for a drink here or a cigarette or the joys of the pub. Sharna doesn't annoy me anymore. She's as unreal as me.

Sometimes after the shock therapy you feel robbed of your thought processes and dream-impulses, the desire to daydream is the oldest thing of delight in me, to captivate and thank the divine and thankfulness of love.

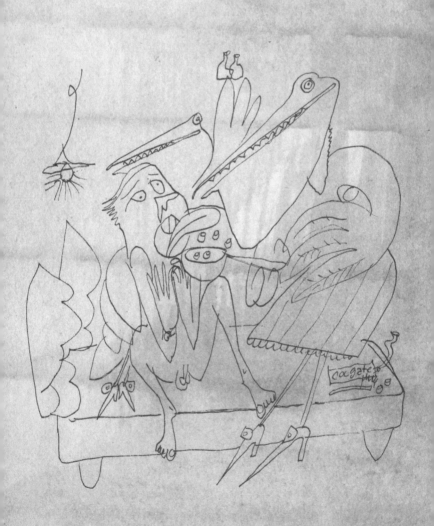

Chapter
nine

I'VE GROWN ACCUSTOMED to the Unit on the third floor of unreality.

Some of the patients actually fear leaving. They dread it. It is all they speak of as they confer in corners: the terror of reuniting with their families in suburbia. And fair enough when you consider what suburbia looks and feels like. Like one big Unit.

It is an unnatural but at the same time crazy community one becomes part of, and distant from, should you fail to understand whether it is real or unreal depending on one's sensations at the time. One is desperate to get out and reacquaint oneself with sweet morning strolls and breakfast with one's family and going to and from work – God, how I need to go back to the workforce again – whatever that is. The mere sight of the nurses may prove distressing, even nauseating, but you need them to get back. They're the key.

The drugs are spooned into us like mother birds feeding their young, even the gaping mouths of the ill can make you want to scream or withdraw into opaqueness.

I like the colossus Kevin, who is articulate and knowledgeable and handsome in his bipolar way; he is a much wittier speaker than the morose others, so amusing and quick with his observations you wonder why he's here. He is a stand-up and a voracious reader and has studied the various philosophies of Carl Jung and Sigmund Freud and Premier Brumby. He is just as comfortable speaking about cubism as psychoanalytical euphemisms. He has a huge head of auburn curly hair and this strong, massive frame so that he resembles Atlas without fuss, like he could be a winning weightlifter at the Beijing Games or some sort of indefatigable wrestler no one could come to grips with, this enormous six-foot man who is so very scared of all kinds of things. But he is given to bouts of sudden flaming rage and his face instantly switches from peace to war. He is unforgiving in regard to assumed slights, and punches the canteen table with his enormous fists so the cutlery rattles upsettingly and unpredictably and dishes vibrate and soup splashes over the rim. You can imagine him pulling a log like an elephant in a waterhole.

'I swing both ways all the time from peace to war,' he sneers as he sips his broth in a dainty way with his little pinkie out like in the Edwardian etiquette books. 'I don't know what it is I am so angry about nor why I am so blissful a half second later. A person's inquiring glance can conquer me or some insignificant thing someone in a shop says just as a throwaway comment can put me into such a completely wrathful condition I can hardly bear it and there are no tablets for that kind of quick change when you are in public.'

He is in for weeks or months, not as long as me, but weeks here is long all right, no matter how you look at it. He doesn't have ECT as I do but perhaps he should because his anger seems unmanageable. You can't imagine him in a shop or behind a counter selling paperbacks in a jovial and wise way, wrapping up the latest Thomas Keneally novel and saying, 'Have a good day!' He is so big with such a staggering body mass you can't imagine him in his bed. He'd be bigger than it. He's to lie on it with his huge muscular legs way over its edge and his size fifty sandshoes bigger than the door of his sombre room filled with books he memorises.

He rubs his face with bottled-up action and sighs a lot in the canteen as he tucks into crumbed piles of cutlets and mountains of roasted pumpkin and boiled spuds, a veritable feast for an entire tribe of bipolar patients. He is the only one I can really talk to, Kevin, and he makes me laugh, really chuckle at his witticisms and drolleries. He's an angry Droll.

Post-It time again and Doctor Gilbertson's astonishing put-downs.

Australian depression has never been in better shape. Kids and the old folks in the nursing home all overdosing in perfect harmony. I complain to the psychiatrist that the wooziness I feel with all the medication he's put me on, insisted upon, his continuous increase of daily drugs is making me feel just terrible.

'In what way, terrible?'

In every way conceivable, terrible.

'Yesterday you claimed it was too hot in the clinic here, yet no other patient made a similar accusation. You also claimed the medication you are taking made you feel giddy, but no one else says they feel that way. You also said your legs felt like flubber!'

By God, he's doing my voice back to me. He's impersonating my whinge.

He is actually raising his voice. I think he's the one who's got anger management concerns, but of course he keeps a firm lid on it. He flips open his wheel-along, collapsible, pitch-black vinyl writing desk to get his hooks on his endless exercise books of close handwriting about my psychotic condition. He never bends over his handwriting, but sits nice and ramrod straight to enter his observations and to quote me.

'Why were you so distressed last night? Rhonda found you

out on the balcony in an anguished state and alerted your state to other night-staff.'

I was too hot, the air-conditioning had altered and it was making me feel clammy and claustrophobic, you know?

'Not really.'

Well, I was so hot and found it difficult to catch my breath and generally the names being called out so loudly on the PA system late at night disturbs me.

'Are you a light sleeper?'

Well, of course I am. I went into St Vincent's in the first place due to chronic insomnia, that's what started my heavy depression, that was the beginning of my illness, the nightly guarantee of no sleep, then driving off to teach in schools filled up with Nescafé to try to keep up; the whole thing made me so jittery and uncertain of myself.

'Oh? I thought it was due to the separation, that the marriage break-up, the failure of your marriage caused your admission into hospital.'

Well, it didn't make me feel any better. I don't want to separate.

'But she has put the separation in train?'

Yes, she has. She wants divorce.

'And you don't?'

No, I still love her.

'Even though she has told you to your face she doesn't love you?'

Yes.

'But it's a bit unreasonable, isn't it, what you want?'

I suppose love has always been unreasonable.

'Your wife insists upon ECT for you because she is exhausted by your life as a vegetable, a man posing as a vegetable.'

You're insulting me.

'Not at all. All you do is lie in your bed and vegetate, you never help in the home, you consume vast quantities of wine at four o'clock in the afternoon and chainsmoke cigarettes and then take a relaxing bath while your exhausted hard-working wife does all the run-around, collecting your son from school, ironing the clothes, stacking the freshly washed clothes away, peeling the potatoes and cooking the schnitzel.'

I work hard at my writing.

'I don't think you do a single thing.'

I never requested an interrogation.

'Maybe you need to strongly contemplate exactly what it has to be like to live with you? I think your wife got tired of your vegetation years ago, but due to her kindness she didn't wish to hurt your feelings, so she put your divorce on the backburner, leave it for another day kind of thing. Why do you lie in your bed 24/7?'

It isn't any fun being depressed so you get carried away with the power of the negativity of it, you plug your mind into the negativity and turn right off life, you can't help it, you remember lovemaking and when your marriage was loving and sex was erotic, but now she isn't interested and there are no hugs or kisses.

'Why should there be those when you don't earn any of them? You lie in your lazy bed and run a long afternoon bath and do nothing and then demand sexual intercourse from a woman who is down on her knees from sheer exhaustion, who does all the shopping, takes proper care of your child, pays for his education out of her modest salary, buys all of his clothes and entertains him by escorting him sometimes to films, makes sure he's reading the kinds of books he loves, reads to him at night, tucks him in and says goodnight while you lie there doing absolutely nothing but vegetating.'

No, I don't think it's right. I don't know what's wrong with me.

'You just don't want to work, that's all.'

I'm working on a new comedy for the theatre. Have you ever heard of the theatre? I'm manic-depressive and only recognise that term, not bipolar or trauma or flashback, I have always swung vigorously between tragic and comic, like a lot of comedians throughout modern history, because it's so hard writing amusingly and tragically without being trite or derivative. Why don't you google me?

'What makes you think you're funny? What is vaguely funny about you? I haven't seen you smile in all the time you've been in the Unit.'

Look, this relationship between you and me has become nothing but a fight. I need good counselling and proper guidance, not criticism like your put-downs.

'I can't breathe properly, you claim. My body is like flubber, you say all the time. I can't sleep even with the sleeping tablets. My wife wants separation soon as I get out of hospital. Yet she visits you two times out of each working week, doesn't she? With your little boy, Louis, doesn't she? Why do you find so much fault in your honest wife?'

You're taking her side. You're biased and therefore you're against me. You never ever buoy me or even momentarily cheer me up. The first thing you said yesterday to me was you're deteriorating.

'You *are* deteriorating, it may have to do with your blood pressure so I'm going to increase your Micardis intake. Are you taking your nightly Micardis tablets?'

I can't remember. They all look alike.

'It's just so crucial that you never forget to take the medication correctly. Your wife confessed to me over the telephone yesterday morning that you often skip your prescription tablets and just don't take any of them, that you don't even know where they are, that she darts round Melbourne all the time filling in your prescriptions, waiting in line after her work is over and driving home in peak traffic only to discover that again you are just lying in bed without having taken them.'

I've only been like this a few months. I don't know what I'm doing. I'm very sick. How can I explain loneliness to you?

'But the serious fact is you've been off your medication for years, haven't you? That you like to make it hard for your wife. You can't be bothered taking a few pills because you might get better and you like lying in bed doing nothing all day.'

I've got a screaming headache.

'No, you haven't.'

He stares incredulously at me in Interview Room 2. In a minute he'll be gone, vanished with his wheel-along impromptu writing desk to hurriedly converse with certain nurses at the nurses station, rapidly gesticulating, rapid eye movements, gleaming pate and clipped nose hairs, violently clipped are those nose hairs that don't stand a single chance of blooming into a full hair of an inch long.

He has completely exhausted me so I walk achingly back to my room and have to lie down, despite all his admonishments about my lying down. I'm not lazy, just sick, that's all. The very second my buggered brain hits the hard cell-block-type pillow that I have to fight each night to get to troubled sleep, Rhonda enters the room and angrily slaps her hands with a loud bang and says this won't do, time for some exercise, you can't just lie there all day doing nothing!

You can't win.

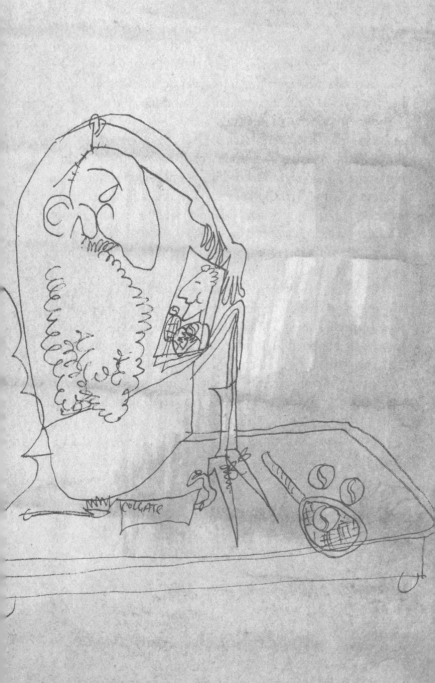

Chapter
ten

EACH EVENING IN THE insane asylum I examine a picture of my little boy. The photograph is normal-enough looking, taken possibly by my friendly wife or my father or one of my brothers at some kind of family gathering, maybe a birthday party. In it I am conversing or listening to a voice outside the image and the mood of the photograph is not so much friendly as protective, with my right arm, suntanned and muscular without the Tarzan quality of superhuman power, but just a contented father of fifty-eight years or thereabouts, with his son who is not so much smiling as perfectly at peace. This old peace in him is not imposed or imagined but genuine. He has been this way ever since my wife gave him life nearly fourteen years ago; he's perhaps six in the snapshot. Angelic and down to earth.

It's the only picture outside my memory of my boy and I am careful with it; very. I nightly look at it before the drugs kick in, particularly the Seroquel, which are so strong that if I swallow a pair of them I just about have to run to bed, they work so fast. And in that running I know full well that I shall be unconscious immediately, that there shall be no insomnia nor sudden accursed wakefulness. They work upon the instant. They might possibly be heroin by another name for all I know.

After millennia of sleeplessness, the Seroquel are my new friends; you only require one of them to sleep in a profound stupor. With a pair of them in you it is rather like being unalive. My nights are memory in Room 5 at the Unit. I called it Ward yesterday with my psychiatrist/interrogator David Gilbertson, who was quick to point out I got the title wrong.

'It's actually Unit,' he said, looking straight through me.

I go to bed like the sick old frightened man I have become.

The sheets are awful, everything is; it is simply horrid to the touch here. No one to kiss you goodnight, no one to laugh with, no one to smile at you through the indifferent dark.

Just his image in the three-year-old Polaroid. This sweet creation who adlibs precisely like his amusing mother. The brilliance and joking and unteachable wisecracking. He's a clown in a world running out of them at a rapid rate. Even with the six strong drugs they've got me on, sometimes I wake up at 2 am. Wide awake and filled with sleeping tablets and high blood pressure capsules and unpronounceable milligrams of gloominess. I wander dreamwise in my underpants and T-shirt through the corridors trying hard to believe I'm here. Every night, all alone I go walking through a vortex.

I'm very nearly sixty and ought to be typing a novel in the suburbs. Sipping tea and giving my blood to the needy. I ought to be dining with Sylvia Plath. Life after forty years of writing should be calm and comfortable and moreish. But here I am in this idiotic psychiatric hospital being insulted every morning. I asked the psychiatrist yesterday to interview me later in the day from now on, claiming I was too medicated to speak properly at 7 am.

He replied, 'That's about all the time we have today, Barry,' and left, wheeling his vaudeville pneumatic writing desk with him, looking just preposterous, but not to anyone else but me, the silent witness of my own burial.

It could easily be five in the morning or three in the afternoon as I walk through the meaninglessness of the Unit. The snoring others, the drugged others so stuffed full of life-reduction tablets. How do I rouse any of them to rouse me? I'm rouseless.

There is this baffling woman called Anne with all this frizzy white and grey matted hair and an acquiline nose; she unfailingly wakes me up at one in the morning by holding a great big square torch before her scrawny body and when I sit bolt upright and complain that she has again woken me she replies, 'Just doing the rounds.' The rounds involves persecuting the doped patients by waking them up all the time and counting them. Even the carpet feels inhuman here, with vinyl dust motes floating up out of them as you pass. The loneliness of vinyl dust motes is all we are. Jesus Christ, I'm literally turning into Sylvia Plath. I've always wanted to write as well as she did.

My wife and my son: are they coming to see me today or tonight? It has to be tonight as she has a full-time job as a Catholic Primary School Teacher in the suburbs. It must be hard to drive after work in peak traffic to pick up our boy from his school then drive the extra kilometres through aggro, choked traffic to call in to see me. She always looks exhausted because she actually always is. She gives me ironed pants and there is nothing to say.

We have our family meal in the hospital canteen and they are both starving so I watch them tuck into the grilled chicken and baby potatoes and sip their lemonade and my wife looks up with a weary grin and says, 'It's so much easier to eat here after so long a day teaching.' Her hip is killing her. She winces when she gets up. Everything's an effort.

My son and I play table tennis in a joyous sort of way in the Recreation Room, he is brilliant at all ball games and hits each ball with an eagerness and pleasure that blooms with each passing forehand. She watches us play and claps and laughs and I start thinking, you know, why don't we stay together as a family; we get on great most of the time, but the truth is we have fought each other too much. Too many recriminations. Two clowns out of touch.

And as she says herself so acutely, indeed it's a favourite saying of hers, 'You can never take the bitter words back again; they hang in the air and are there forever.' Only a Catholic could say or think that. I've always felt we could love again. Always.

They depart again and I see them to her station wagon and tell her to drive carefully and my son waves goodbye to me again and as they head off I stare at their back indicator light winking on and off and now they are completely gone. It's only seven o'clock at night and there's nothing of any kind to do except keep getting medicated.

There being nothing to do, I come back to bed again and look at my little boy Lou. I want to hold him, hold my wife, but we don't do that anymore. I think about separation and her recent note of goodbye. 'It's hard for you to contemplate separation in the midst of the horrors of ECT.'

It isn't that hard; it's impossible.

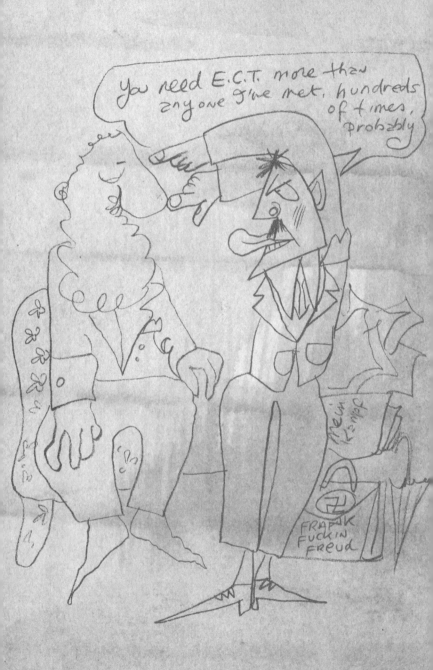

Chapter
eleven

THE NEXT ECT IS scheduled for 7 am today. I feel the same. Awful. Awfuller, actually. As usual the four of them arrive like Ku Klux Klan psychiatric nurses. Silhouetted in black but wearing white, stark is the white they wear. The Anne one bearing a torch shining it right into my eyes. One beckoning me to follow. We move towards the lift well and one silently pushes the lift button to descend. There is no need of talk and no need of comfort. The big new steel and chromium lift jerks to a shuddering halt. We walk like men in a posse.

I am gestured to sit. So I indeed sit on a very hard pink armchair that doesn't even hiss when I sit in it. You cannot get comfortable in this thing, no matter how hard you wriggle and fidget. It is of course with a sense of suspended disbelief that I am going ahead with this. My wife wants me to have it and is being pressured to agree with it by the psychiatrist. I don't want it but have no soul to call my own so just put up with it each time. I can't blame them for trying anything on me.

I can see a patient out of TS Eliot, etherised upon a cloud or table. His or possibly her limbs hang down off it lifelessly and stark whitely. There is absolutely no sound in here. Just, if you can imagine it, the sound of waste.

When shall it be my turn? inquires the conscience. I merely sit there blankly and wait for over an hour feeling not so much afraid as dull. Dulled by the boredom of electroconvulsive paranoia.

The door is ajar and Ian the horrible grinning eunuch folk-guitar bastard is assisting an old person to get up on the etherising table and strap on the smoky yellowish gas mask. I very much wish to vomit. If I did they'd do it to me anyway, I guess, awash with sick; they wouldn't postpone. They never put off anything.

A young boy is given it and the door is wide open by now so I can look right in. He looks about twenty or thereabouts and he is given the injection and the gas. I feel as if I'm living in the fifteenth century. Why don't they give me a block of wood to bite into?

The team of electrocutionists never say 'Hi!' to the new ECT patient or even wave to them or show any sign of recognition. It's just one after the other; then back to bed to recover, sleep it off all day. The sycophantic Ian greases to all the patients in a never-ending display of pseudo-friendliness and false-Christian bonhomie. I actually can't stand him, but like all terrible events in life you simply have to. He will go away and I will recover and that will be the end of Ian. I realise you're not to hate but that is the only possible emotion I feel towards Ian. As if to kill him. Because of his greasy perpetual grin. I wonder what on earth is he now grinning at? Me. He's grinning at me because he is to give me ECT. He's a gargoyle and a sycophant pig.

On the preparation table I hop and feel as though I'm to be embalmed. My mother gave me life and now they steal it and waste me and betray me with all their confounding electrical wizardry. One of the nurses injects a short silver needle in my left wrist and I am instantly unconscious. The other nurse puts on the gas mask and presses it on me. 'Just breathe naturally,' she intones, looking bored stupid. They put the stink-smelling green gel in my hair and the tapes go on the nape of my neck now. They administer a small electric jolt to lift my mood. I feel awful.

My eyes are sore, my back hurts me and my arms really ache a great deal all of a sudden. I can't recall if I walked alone back to my bed in Room 5 or got there by wheelchair. In the event I am depressed and back in bed. Is my mood lifted or my mind stolen temporarily or possibly permanently?

Barry has five drugs per evening that offer addiction but not help. My general practitioner recommends my weaning myself off them but does not say how. I take two enormous Efexor that are for depression; does that mean they give depression to you?

I take one thiamine tablet to make up for decades of alcoholism. Am I an alcoholic? I suppose so. I mean I feel like one. Is a bottle every three nights an alcoholic? Probably I'm not. I never miss drink.

I take one Micardis tablet for my heart, which is full of love for my son.

I take one Ostelin tablet for Christ knows what.

What I liked, what was so cute about my psychiatrist was the heartfelt manner in which he praised these drugs, speaking of them in awe and wonder, in a truly reverent way. And that is true also of the nurses on duty at the medication window at eight at night, handing out powerful addictive drugs with styrofoam beakers filled with tap water to the doped.

The whole system is full of fantastic contradictions. On the one hand they are to bring you back to life; on the other they are to drug you and give you shock therapy that no one in Australia and possibly the world still believes goes on in clinics for mental health. And yet it is on the rise. Thousands swear by it.

Anne the stunted, humped-over witch with the mop of wispy, stiff grey shoulder-length hair holds the square metallic torch on me again at exactly two in the morning and I have swallowed a palm full of strong antidepressants and am groggy.

'Just doing a head-count,' she shrieks as she always does, in a very curt manner. You cannot reply to a sentence like that one. You wake up and feel awful all the time; then you are told you require more tablets to lift your mood. I assume I shall be in here forever. I *was* there forever. Six months of going nowhere.

Do NOT Resist E.C.T you bastard Dickins

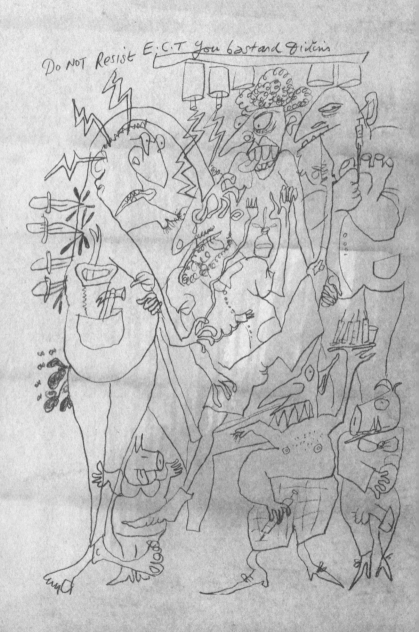

Chapter
twelve

MY HANDS TREMBLE so badly I cannot hold a pen to write, to capture anything. I have several blank pages of paper ripped out of a notebook but can't write with so trembly a writing hand; even when I'm endeavouring to eat fried rice in the canteen it goes everywhere, spilling on the floor and marking my pants with spilt soy, the worst smell in the world that is. I abhor soy.

But the eating of food was pushed well beyond the human limit as well as the unquestioning regard to gulping tablets. One morning Sharna chased me into my room with a heaped-up plate of Greek salad that was at least half a day over its use-by limit, and she leapt like a quivering she-devil onto my bed – usually a safe haven – and tried to ram it down my throat. I'm being force-fed.

Her face was transported, it was somewhere other than sensible, she screamed at me to such a degree I could see into her head through the raging, inflamed tonsils. I could see her gizmos rolling around their bizarre circuitry.

'You *have* to eat this! This will sustain you! Open your mouth! How do you expect to lift your mood if you refuse to eat!' I have always hated Greek salad, that's why I'm not enthused about it. Sharna won't acquiesce; she holds a gigantic forkful of revolting fetta with gooey tomato hooked onto it and fronds of trendy suntanned lettuce and spirals of ugly spring onion, enough to feed an army of depressives, and pantomimes my teeth penetrating all of it, with almost tears of exasperation she says with the utmost force of will, 'Will you eat your nutrition or not!'

Not. I'm a very wilful boy.

It tumbles in its own bowl to the vinyl carpet on my floor where all the other bits of forced meals have fled to; oh well, they shall have to vacuum.

I peer into this strange nurse entitled Sharna. She is most definitely Malaysian. She is not attractive in any sort of way; she is masculine-looking and forceful and dominating as though she were once the court executioner. 'You are literally starving yourself to death!' she gargles and her forehead is all tightly drawn and painful-looking wrinkles so that I start to feel empathy for her, not to mention concern for her health. She needs antidepressants. The planet earth does.

I explain to her that for decades I've been an overweight writer, due no doubt to all the fish and chips and pies and sauce and sausage rolls to keep me rhyming. Junk food is excellent for your alliteration. Eventually she admits temporary defeat and slinks out in a marked way back to the nurses station.

'Barry Dickins to the nurses station,' comes the ear-shattering new announcement.

Surely they have made some kind of a mistake. I have never been summoned before, so why now, at this moment? They tell me off for borrowing another patient's mobile to make a rapid call to my wife and son. 'You cannot keep pressuring other patients who are in here suffering from advanced stress!' they point out at the top of their voices in a deafening cacophony of negativity. So what about a local call? So what about them at the idiotic nurses station?

It is the pecking orders that really get you down in a psychiatric institution like this. The nurses never miss a trick, due to boredom mixed with not being educated. If I am trying to borrow a trendy mother's mobile to make a call they are instantly onto it and tell me off in front of everyone to embarrass me. 'There's no use in upsetting Sylvia, is there, Barry? You obtain your own mobile and never mind borrowing them from already distraught fellow patients.'

That's blackmail, I think. Everyone's distraught.

One of my many visitors to this clinic is old friend, book editor Bruce Sims, who attended the same high school I failed at, Merrilands in Keon Park. Bruce lost his nose to cancer so wears a false one bravely enough and still smokes all the time, luxuriously exhaling through both vinyl nostrils.

Soon he shall have all his teeth removed as his gums have been affected by radiotherapy. No one could have it rougher than he, surely, yet here he is sitting so placidly upon my bed clasping his hands so gently like a peaceful man does talking to me. He swings his legs in glee whenever he chuckles, raspy and often are those chuckles of his, the twinkling eyes and never-say-die expression. He is a good storyteller and it isn't so long before we are both in fits of raucous laughter; mostly to do with publishing gossip and writers' gossip. Even Jesus was a gossip. That's what the bible mostly is. Gossip. It separates us from the oh-so-bored crypt.

I couldn't believe it when he walked in; in the condition he's in and the worry that must be in his mind and memory of when he was just fine. With all that unstoppable energy and charisma and unstoppable love of new writing.

He edited my second memoir, published by Penguin, entitled *I Love to Live*. It appeared in 1991 and sold 5000 copies, which is not bad in Australia. I just wrote a chapter a day and left it with Maria who runs a milk bar over the road from Bruce, and

Maria inserted each typed recollection in her icecream freezer for Bruce to edit when he came in to buy his smokes. It worked like a charm.

He edited the snap-frozen prose as he chainsmoked at his editing desk. Next day I would obviously turn up and give dear Maria chapter two or possibly the artwork for the wrap-around cover and she would look at it critically and squint her eyes at it then put it in a no-fuss way among the frozen vegies: broccoli and carrots and what have you. I wrote the book in a careless and disciplined way, you'd have to say a frozen happy way.

To write elegantly you call it fun, rather like a slide in the park. I've never had a bother with writing. Only life.

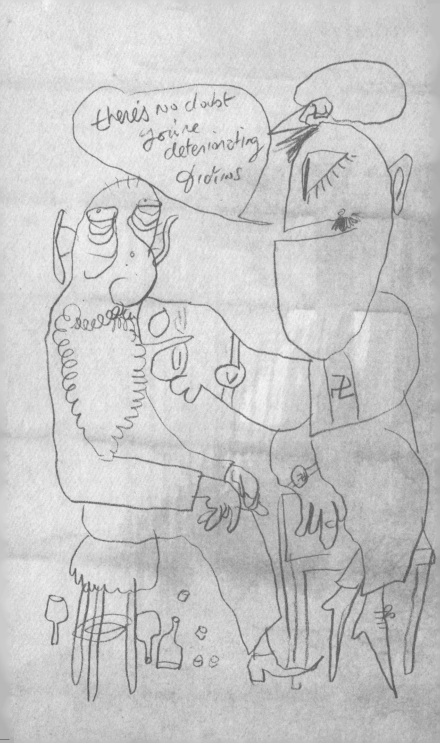

Chapter
thirteen

THE 7 AM INTERROGATIONS do you not a whit of good. He smiles in the old familiar way as though we haven't seen each other for at least a day. Has it been a day? It seems less – more like a second.

'Do you know where you are?'

Yes, the Ward.

'Actually, it's a Unit.'

Fair enough.

'You talk in an old-fashioned sort of a way, don't you think? I mean who uses that colloquialism "Fair enough" anymore?'

I don't know.

'Do you know today's date?'

No.

'Don't you remember today's date?'

I'd rather have a date scone.

'What do you remember of your latest ECT?'

Nothing.

'Because of your years of heavy alcohol consumption we are increasing your thiamine intake to two capsules of them a day; and also increasing your vitamin A intake. There's no doubt your frontal lobes have been extensively damaged. What did you drink each day? One bottle of white wine per day and a couple of stubbies, wasn't it, in your courtyard in Carlton?'

Often as not. One night a week. No more than one night.

'What, more than one bottle and a few stubbies in the courtyard?'

I didn't always drink in the courtyard. But only one night a week.

'You drank wherever you found yourself, then?'

Yes. I found myself at least one night a week.

'Didn't you realise that would do you a great deal of harm over decades of abuse, that this is the real cause of your clinical depression, your sleeplessness, your tinnitus probably?'

The tinnitus was caused by living on a main road with billions of semi-trailers screaming on it; it felt as if they were coming right through the bedroom walls.'

'Isn't that a bit of an exaggeration, isn't that an exaggerated thing to say?'

How much have you written about me in biro? Are you having it published?

'I have to keep a case history on your improvement in the Unit. You have drunk too much over the decades and now you're bottoming out; why do you vegetate at your terrace home your wife has ordered a renovation for, why do you think you never get up out of your bed, but are perfectly content to just lie there and rot?'

I don't rot deliberately, doctor. It's an illness, that's why I'm here in your care. You're the one guilty of exaggeration.

'You've been in my care for six weeks and yet you're no better than when you signed yourself in; do you have any fear of being released? Some psychiatric patients are actually very distressed about the concept of going back to their homes, did you know that?'

Perhaps their homes are more distressing than being a patient here, perhaps their own family destroys them, don't love them there and never miss a single chance to point that fact out, that they are loathed and held beneath their so-called loved ones' contempt. I can identify with that fear but I myself don't personally feel it.

'Are you certain of that fact or just assume this is your actual opinion? You and your wife have had terrible fights early this year, which don't spring out of nowhere but out of your laziness.'

I never stop working. I had two exhibitions of my paintings at the same time in January, one in Hampton and another in Bundoora; that was a retrospective exhibition and those exhibitions were a lot of work, incredible energy went into each of them and we had an enormous fight, my wife and I, on the evening before my first retrospective, so that I attended it on my own which is an intensely depressing thing to do as an artist.

'What difference would it make if your wife couldn't get there? Do you expect her to support everything you do?'

More than half of my paintings are celebrations of my feelings towards my wife.

'But you can't in all conscience demand that she be there every single time you exhibit yourself, can you? Isn't that placing unfair expectations upon her, when you think about it?'

I had to make a speech at my retrospective without her being there; it was difficult for me to keep smiling with her somewhere else after a lifetime of painting. In a sense we painted everything together.

'How did the speech go?'

It went over all right but it would have been much better if she'd been there.

'Even if you were hating each other?'

It wasn't so much hate as not getting on. There's an enormous difference between hating and just niggling.

'But you never get on. Even though she comes in to see you every second night now you're having electroconvulsive therapy.'

She's very good at visiting people when they're stuck in hospital.

'Is that how you see yourself? As stuck?'

And so the interrogation goes, on and on interminably until he tells me that's about all the time he has for me this morning, Barry. He always concludes each session with, 'That's all the time we have today, Barry.' I watch him go about the show business of folding up the portable wheel-along-desk-cum-trolley-thing, black like his black suit, everything about him is that colour, black, and he whisks away like a mechanical rodent.

I repair to the disillusioning canteen where the others are preparing to chainsmoke in the swirly courtyard; that disillusions me too the way they so furiously chainsmoke, all red in the face and raving away about any old thing during another vile tempest. I prise open a miniature box of Just Right cereal, which I've become addicted to, and add plenty of sugar as I need plenty of sugar after each interview with him in either Interview Room 1 or Interview Room 2. I patiently tip longlife milk upon the bizarre box of grainy flakes guaranteed to lift my mood. It says so on the packet. I add some oily, disgusting, macabre, pregnant, burpy black prunes hoping to put some closure to my constipation, the only thing to come out of all my hundreds of drugs. I've been utterly blocked since I was admitted. All I do is hiss.

Because of the bright light shafting through the nut-house and the effect of the antidepressants I can't tell the time of day or recall where my horrid room is. I sat on my two-dollar reading spectacles the other day so I can't read a thing except the endless Post-Its adhered to my bureau next to my restless hard hospital bed. I adore them. They're like an Egyptian comic strip.

I flop in one of the TV rooms. There are two of them, and watch the Beijing Olympics as the grinning-at-nothing bipolar patients applaud or boo. The schizophrenic patients watch each sporting event twice – with either great passion or it appals them. The woman who had Day Leave and trooped off to her native trendy Brunswick Street Fitzroy to have a catch-up with her old friends and share her experiences at the Unit, but with a devastating outcome, couldn't handle it. This is the second time.

'I just couldn't handle something I was so looking forward to,' she blubbers as her bipolar tears cascade down her pretty face. 'They couldn't understand why I signed myself in here voluntarily, they all have their lives in order, they don't hallucinate, they think that it's merely in movies or books. I tried so hard to be "up" in their carefree company, but I got panicky instantly and couldn't stand it and caught the tram back here.' Poor bitch is mad like me.

She stares at her meal and half-heartedly plays with the string beans with the back of her dull fork. I wanted to hug her, but of course one doesn't.

At half past eight at night a trendy, tall, elegantly dressed lady of six feet in height with high heels on and her hair up at the back and tons of make-up on comes into the Unit pushing a very costly pram with a newborn baby in it. She looks like the Queen of the Nile. Dead. Is her depression post-natal or some other form of the enveloping sickness that is devouring my country? These drop-dead exquisite corpse new mothers never tire of giving birth to babies who are instantly depressed. They dream-walk each hour into my lift and stare meaningless into disinfected air. I ponder their husbands, their histories, their psychological need to bear sad embryos and see them go to term as fully fledged schizophrenics. They resemble an army of erotic deceased depressives whose working husbands come in at night and fetch their trendy cigarettes, which they light for them in the communal emphysema garden at the rear of the canteen. It is as though postnatal depression is a cult. They must take hours to apply their devastating make-up. Their whispered conversations are laced with nothingness. Just add obliqueness. Are they my fellow man or not? I must say they are surreal and strange-looking, these myopic mums. It's not their fault of course that they're mad. It's no one's fault. We just are here.

The dormant others, the paralysed others, the sick others upset me. How weary you become of their constant complaining, whingeing it is called in my country. The constant criticisms of patients who have chucked life, who jettisoned joy and archived excitement and pointed the bone at natural-born comedy that I swore used to be in us all; now I am not sure it was ever in me. The old passion to be alive.

One day I accepted Day Leave and signed the book at reception and walked two miles into sunny Carlton to meet Aristotle; that's his real name. Paris Aristotle, a human rights advocate who I've been seeing over two years in order to write a book on torture. I'm perfectly placed to write something like this. Interviews with refugees, that sort of thing. I felt redeemed just to be out walking instead of being in and going nowhere. I love walking around Melbourne. I've been doing it for fifty-eight years now.

The feet still worked, so did the arms and back. I got out of there for a while and forsook the ECT. I had a toasted sandwich with Paris who has got a very big, bald head but a very charming manner, and it wasn't long before he was talking passionately about how his son plays soccer and I was speaking about how good my son is at tennis, how he plays for Fitzroy with his team-mates.

I walked all the way back up St Kilda Road and thought about how good it felt to laugh again with someone ordinary. I felt terrible going back into the ward for the unwell, often the deliberately unwell. I hate being sick and down.

I managed to keep my diary going when in the clinic, my work diary that is, but my hand shook too much for me, the rest of me that is, to write using it. I used to perch in my chair next to my hospital bed and smile in a bemused way I suppose and look at my hand trembling so much and wonder why that was. It shook due to my nerves being shot. No doubt.

I know I hallucinated about two months into my stay. My friend Tom Gelai and his son Hugo came to visit me and we were out in this front balcony, like a nuclear sitting room where the brain-damaged chatted to their meek or barbaric families away from the madding crowd.

I assumed the clinic was on fire in some way and couldn't stand the heat of it; I asked Tom to ask a minor official to ask a fireman to turn the heat down to normal, but Tom said someone said it *was* normal, but the air-conditioning didn't work properly, that was clear to me, and I remember I marched like a fatigued soldier up and down the corridor for ages in complete despair that everything was too hot. I know that I kept on muttering all the time.

After Tom and his child were gone I slept drugged straight away in my favourite body-position, dead chap. The colossal rates of sleep fixed me. The deep sleep treatment, for such it was, cured me. For decades I'd been awake and isolated in the centre of my closest friend, the night. The dreadful dilemma of not knowing how to relate to Tom and his son drove me to feeble-minded horror. I'd become a paranoid mute.

I realised as soon as Tom had gone and I was alone in my room that it was a perfect echo of my mother's hallucination, that nothing was of comfort, let alone the family, who were as strange as your own strangled voice. I had always been scornful of her madness and now I too was insane. Perfectly.

In the morning I breakfasted with the insane others on cereals and fresh milk, though I didn't peruse the newspaper, because none were delivered for us penitents, and the slovenliness and the occasional dignity of the eaters was a sort of abstract communion and a sort of family, I suppose. But the closer I became to them the more lost I truly felt inside my hide. I didn't want their friendship or their interest – especially not their trust.

I am escorted for my next ECT at precisely six-thirty in the morning Eastern Summer Time and am merely a frightened old father with a very white beard and pot gut and false teeth, separated at birth from beauty. They don't bother to say anything this time as we've all been through it before, lots. Is this my sixth torture?

Descend the awful lift and plod over to the bad-taste armchairs and sit uncomfortably upon one of them waiting to be zapped.

There is no thought nor sound just the deed of getting it again in the human-being head. As you so meekly and thoroughly comply with the obscenity of electrocuting your mind, your poet's mind, you often feel the jig is up. That the most depressing aspect of clinical surrender is your own compliance. Your dumb meekness. You who are no longer, you have agreed to agree with someone you instinctively loathe. Your profession assessor/psychiatrist keeps on insisting that ECT shall lift your mood. It and it alone shall lift your misbegotten mood: which I say is your soul itself. Is there anything wrong with being down-in-the-dumps?

The saddest aspect of one's own downfall, one's tragedy that it has bottomed out and come to this is that there is no one to talk to about it. One's wife can't mind too much that you are terrified of having it so often; I couldn't believe it when as a post-mortem, after I got out, she confessed to me in her car that I'd had it nine times; I thought it was six times. She didn't care that I was frightened going into it and coming out of it because she was to leave me. I couldn't blame her one jot.

Prone on the drugged table where so many other Melburnians have been is a particular helplessness I need to record as a poet. You feel contempt for them, the grim automatons who dully administer the convulsion that robs you of your identity, to lift your invisible spirit as he never ceases to tell me. I hate his chastising and constantly enfeebling voice.

His Trinity College voice is superior to my Keon Park voice. He is always impatient and never listens to me and I am a raconteur; speaking on the ABC is something I've done to pay the mortgage, part-pay the mortgage that is, when I was happily married. And that was for twenty years at least.

It is his indefatigable droning that wears my spirit right down to the stumps. Just having to look at him each morning wears me out. He is to kill me; that is how I feel in my drugged brain, the administering of enormous capsules that contain my death.

The cheerful way the nurses administer them to the never-questioning patients. I hate their meekness. Are they all Christians?

The vomit of having no say. The nausea of giving up on responses. The nothingness a husband feels upon reading the wife's letter of farewell in one's hospital bed. It is not her fault and I know I am impossible to live with due to too passionate a spirit and too raucous a personality but she is a kindred raucous personality and lately says she is seeking counselling and is mixed up as I am mixed right up upon the separation she instigated.

The hardest thing about ECT is the complete isolation of one's impending loneliness of the spirit. It is for the surrendering poet's gloom that they perform it upon what is left of you. You tell no one and remember nothing. They cast you in a briskly driven wheelchair after it and rush you back to your stupid bed again to live longer.

My honest old father who is ninety wrote me a letter I treasure and keep in the clutter of my writing desk; in it he speaks of wondering if any of the doctors and psychiatrists are aware that I have won the Premier's Award for Drama or the International Amnesty Award for Peace through Art. Of course not. Only a man who loves his son could compose a letter like that. Oh, how much more intelligent is my old father than the people here who claim they are to help us back to life. They only help us back to more loneliness and drug addiction. They need Len Dickins here badly.

Nary a patient here would ever say to a nurse, 'Oh, by the way, you are wrong there,' or perhaps, 'No thanks, I don't want my daily medication increased.' You are immediately nothing. You cannot even have or possess your own thoughts in your bed as they are constantly asking you how you are getting on; and of course you have absolutely no idea of that, so how could you tell them anything about anything? You munch your lowbrow cereal and shut your milk-rammed face. Their treatment is your sickness.

For some reason it is the morning cereal in miniature boxes and the free milk that give my day here any modicum of meaning; the familiarity of television ads promoting blinding boxes of Special K or Corn Flakes Now Containing Real Honey that are the only comfort due to the overpowering reality of brainwashing or television nostalgia that makes up all our dumbfound days, that gives us hope and the shits simultaneously. It is rather like being shot in a firing squad and then given glucose to lift your mood.

'Ready, aim, light and crunchy!'

'Ready, aim, Special K!'

After the soporific pep talk from the doctor who has no sense of humour you wander back to bed because there is nowhere else to go but insanity, or the relaxation class given by a mind thief. Disco music and stretch exercises for the decomposing. 'And it's one and two and drop completely dead!'

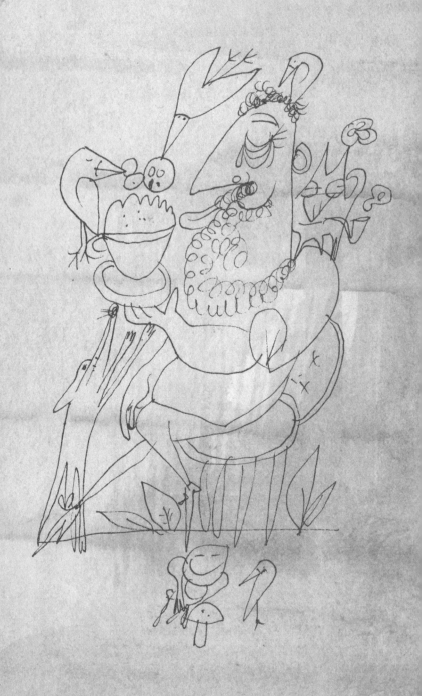

Chapter
fourteen

ONE SPRING AFTERNOON I signed the 'Leave' book, which is the most bureaucratic thing here, for you must write the reason you are leaving, whether it is by foot or car, how long you are leaving and when you estimate you'll return. You could get a cramp filling in the paperwork to go for a nice walk. I signed and strode the city, finding all my favourite trails and ways through green parks, and adored once more to see the last of the old bookshops and cathedrals I worshipped all through my boyhood. I had a nice lunch with an amusing public servant and it felt fantastic to sip coffee that was real and not mechanical and laugh unmechanically. I wanted normality so desperately.

I took my time going back and loved seeing my fellow citizens in the hubbub and natural calamity of crowded streets. Since I grew up in the street and interviewed the street and remembered every syllable spoken there, it felt like vindication to hurtle back into living literature of the footpath. I am a footpath.

How unalive and unwelcoming the clinic was after the hurly burly of walking back to life in the famous brick buildings and incinerated staircases of old post offices, where I'd sorted mail as a teenager. I knew every brick of my hometown and every speech delivered in every street of it; now I am signing the leave book and among the captive and the cautious, the more than meek, the arrogantly afraid. The boastfully bipolar. The machine-mad. The trendy delusional.

It staggered me that so many people in there were dreading going back home; possibly they were mocked and beaten in their homes; more than likely they were unloved in them, as poor Ed the guy who was interfered with by his insane father displayed that night next to the medication dispensary window when he had his violent, covered-up flashback.

My hands shook all the time. The routine of it, the boredom of it, the insatiable desire of the nurses to simultaneously drug you to deepest sleep only to rudely awaken you at two in the morning by performing a head count; shining a goddamned torch into your drugged eyes.

I required the darling buds of May; I wanted to get out of there but I was not so much lethargic as completely flat. That indeed is just what real depression is. It is flat. Like a flat bike tyre. Flat. You eat without taste or appetite and sleep meaninglessly. No matter what you do you feel unloved, unrewarded, ghastly, ghostly, invisible and the nausea of being not so much meek as without form or outline. Your past is a fake and your future is all illusory.

My father, who is eighty-nine and three-quarters and suffers a smorgasbord of health bummers from osteo- and rheumatoid-arthritis and knee failure, so they unscrew whenever he is trying to get up and perambulate as he has perambulated since his mother had him in 1919, his will is considerable, and when he hobbled into my room at the clinic and sat in the visitor's chair with an 'oomph!' effect as his skinny arse sank ever lower, I felt redeemed theatrically and morally. Here was Arlecchino straight out of Commedia dell'Arte. His very entrance was out of *A Servant of Two Masters*. He was Cyrano and Len all together in a fantasy called real recovery. He was better than Seroquel.

He just stared into my drugged blue eyes without love or indifference or judgement or forgiveness but understanding; he understood me because he understood death and I was dead before he gave me life and came in the dead room where they kept me dead without dead hope. The old love of he who gave me existence reared up. Out of the history and the ancestry came joy unparalleled and hope fulfilled in one glance at he who mattered since none of the others did, not a jot.

He pushed the cheap industrial chair across. He wheeled the black and cheap vinyl (everything in the Unit is cheap vinyl) and sat by me, a fourth of his sons; he has never given favour. He doesn't have favourites, not him.

He said with that wrinkly, wise, working-class visage of his, 'When you getting out?' In other words it was up to me. My call. Nothing to do with experts on my condition. That would do it. That was the prompt I required not to stuff up. He meant: 'It's up to you. You can lie here and die or leave and work.' The work was to write this for my only friend, the reader. Put your pants on and leave. So I did.

I made a mental-cognitive note to leave next morning. To check out of the clinic and never return. The other thing that got me out was winning a State Library literary award, the R.E. Ross Trust for Drama. I won $6,100, which seems a rather discursive sum.

That I had won something that had to do with writing made me put my boots on. When the psychiatric nurse handed me the letter from the State Library I made up my mind to quit the clinic and write for my living again; no matter how hard that was, it was better than lying in bed thinking about painting and writing. What could be more meaningless than thinking about what you love to do? Recovery is *doing*, not imagining.

I signed myself out of that hell-hole and recalled a thing said flippantly by Tim, a Cockney psych-nurse of two metres tall who used to sit on my lonesome bed and take notes on my sick mind from time to time over the long weeks I was stuck there. He was an enormous person with doe-sort-of-eyes that went on forever and ever, only to sink into a doughnutty face. 'Don't come back,' was what he said. That was his advice and I took it. I'll never go back to that kind of bastardry.

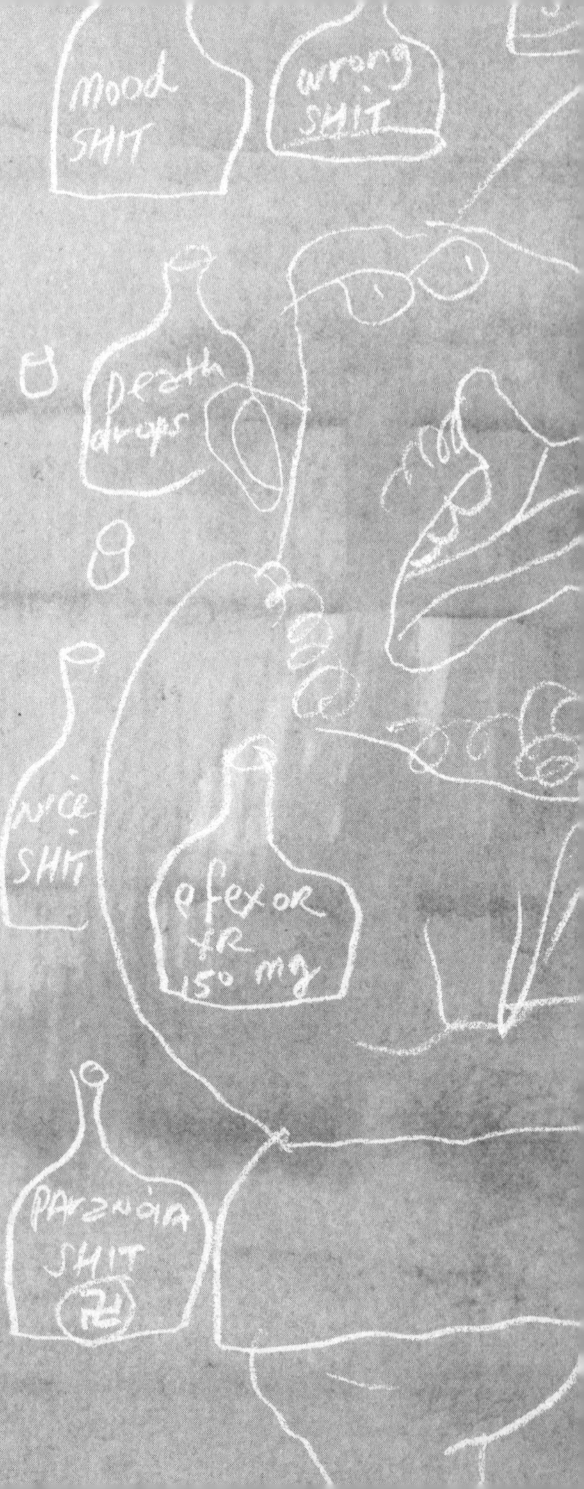
mood SHIT
wrong SHIT
Death drops
nice SHIT
efexor XR 150 mg
Paranoia SHIT

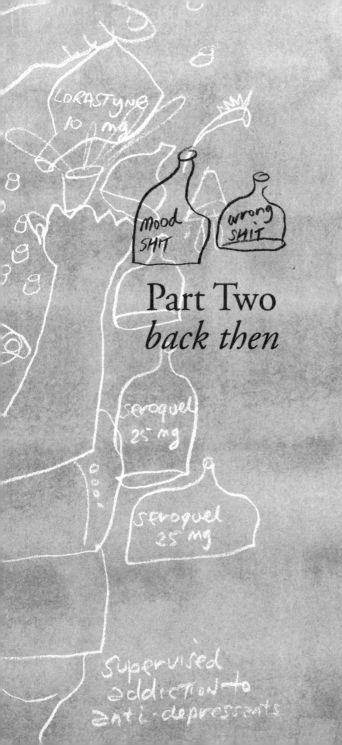

Part Two
back then

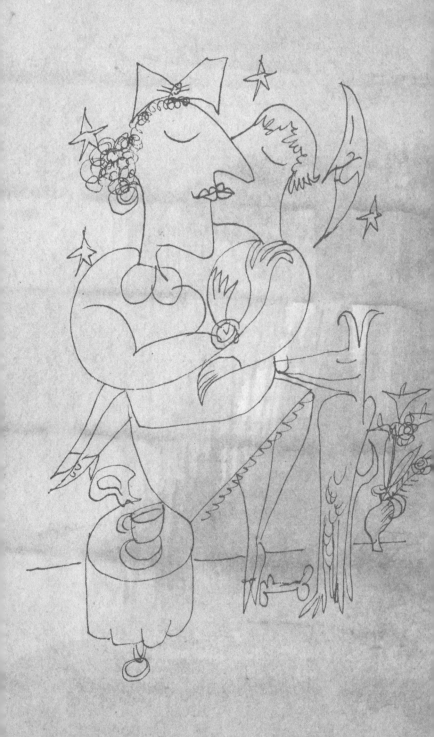

Chapter
one

You REMEMBER ONLY the disasters of your own personal history after ECT. You recall all the failures and disappointments and never the ecstasies and wonders. You remember being insulted and abused verbally by your own family members but not the joy of life and the protracted happiness of being alive: finding yourself alive still after nearly fifty-nine years of bewilderment and overwhelming opening-night excitement.

This is my story of overcoming anxiety and clinical depression all my life. Vincent Van Gogh once wrote, and he was as good a writer as he was a painter, 'Sometimes it's better to be conquered than the conquerer.' And it really is sometimes in the effort to excavate your soul and understand yourself.

The ancestor I'm closest to in character is my paternal grandmother whose Christian name was Gertrude. She lived to be one day off 100. She died of starvation rather than go on with West Preston. When she lay in state at the rear of Ern Jensen's Funeral Parlour in West Preston my father didn't want to observe her and he gave me the evil eye when I did. My brother Rob and I looked at her dead and we both kissed her dead face to take in her passing. She had all these funny shining crystals on her eyelashes.

She was the very essence of obstinacy and bad and good temper which is now called bipolar but then just shittiness. She was shitty to my mum since the day her son went out with her during World War II. She never gave Edna a single chance at independent thought or independent action. She hated her because Edna was so pretty.

The dreadful Christmas day lunches at Gert's place were abominations or stage plays as yet unwritten by Charles Dickens himself, the master satirist who wrote dialogue as his tribe of screechy kids applied jam to his big, bushy beard. My Grandmother Mamie, Edna's mother, who was indomitable, and Gert clashed like Titans as soon as the party started. It was mental warfare and the dry chook choked in your gob. Gert's sister, Bessie Dewhirst, lived there too and they fought even more than Mamie and Gert did, and that's saying something. All of them bipolar grumpies.

Depression amidst families is all about will. The conquerable and unconquerable will to put the other one down for the count. My two grandmothers were both depressed, very. Both lived desperately alone in psychotic ways that delivered paranoia of others as if others were to be frightened of.

Mamie lived solo at 44 Amess Street, Carlton, and although that beautiful, stately, large home with two bedrooms and a dreamy front parlour was hers to relax in and maybe rent out a room, even two to help with the cost of living, she feared others and withdrew into a meek bungalow out the back and slept scared out there, scared of nothing. Everything. Clouds were deliberate trespassers.

The only entertaining Mamie did was to violently and unrelentingly bash her piano in the sitting room, playing to an audience of nobody. She possessed many crumpled, brown and dusty songbooks that were published decades ago with song titles including 'April Showers', 'Mammy' and 'Frosty the Snow

Man'. She accompanied her brutal keyboarding with a fine falsetto whine. She frightened me.

Everything at 'Glastonby', her terrace, was silt: silt upon her dentures and silt upon her windowsills. Silt upon her grey hair and handsome fair face that produced lovely penetrating eyes that grinned at nothing.

Whenever I used to pop in to say 'Hi!' she was assaulting her whimpering piano, the keys rattling away and begging for appeasement, but she *would* play. I pitied her poor old piano.

She was simultaneously glad to see me and displeased. She was a very moody lady who preferred sorrow to joy; I say that since I used to, by chance, see her seated before her vanity mirror in the kitchen, for she put on her make-up in the small kitchen, and, preening, she would make herself tragic by virtue of a whole hour of just staring and eventually tears of sadness would arrive and she'd be pleased with the disastrous effect. 'There – much sadder!'

Preferring loneliness to company she never had anybody in. 'Fuck them.' Her tiny dusty kitchen had autumn leaves in the coffee canisters and her deceased husband Gus's stainless steel oven-ventilation funnels seemed unnecessarily stern to me as a child who sometimes visited. Gus Toll boasted that it was he who invented stainless steel. Sure. In the laundry Gus had bequeathed a steel legacy of stainless taps and stainless faucets and stainless showers and stainless everything. He was stainless indeed because Mamie never mentioned him to me, never.

Mamie invariably had on a brilliantly ironed, hard white apron round her generous waist but never cooked, not a thing. She gardened and developed healthy snail-defiant rows of silverbeet, which she chewed unboiled and direct from the poor plant itself while weeding out there. She was frightened of blacks. 'It's weather for blacks,' she said when it was hot.

The end of Mamie was alarming and exhausting. She was

very badly demented and screamed at things such as car doors opening whenever we endeavoured to hoist her into the rear end of Mum's Charger. She bellyached and carried on like a pork chop. It was difficult to assist her physically because no one really knew what was up with her. We always loved her but that didn't help her mood get up.

My other grandmother, Gert, used to apply twists of brown paper that had soaked overnight in a cup of black tea and then in the new morning she would give hours to the entwining of these twists of paper and tea and then nimbly thread them through her straight whitish hair and after a while, when the West Preston sun showed up at last, her hair went all curly. 'Voila!' So she preferred a homemade afro to traditional boring straight hair, and I have to tell you it looked rather appealing on her honest head. She was pretty, very.

She had the most penetrating blue eyes of anyone I have tried to peer into, in all my years of reporting for newspapers and interviewing or gently interrogating famed persons I have never met an eagle-gaze like hers. She bored straight through me whenever we conversed out the back on her spongy couch grass, which she loved to dive her paws into as she found her words to me. She found the things to say in the very grass she once described as: 'Even this couch grass wants to live.' This said when she lay dying.

Her eyes were blue and huge like the ocean and never appeared once to blink to me sitting by her side on the grass. She possessed a stunning smile got from a goddess whose extraterrestrial bizarreness made me, as a little boy saying 'Hi!' at her doorway, tend to believe she was Mother Mary.

Gert was a gifted listener-to-me-aloud; ever since I can remember she liked me and enjoyed my company. She was so naturally reserved and singular as a daphne bush. She used not to say a thing except, 'What are you up to?' I would then wistfully attempt in my random way to fill in the rest of the spoken text. The wonderful thing was that she didn't judge me. She was my best friend and whenever she went to the fuss of cooking for me when I slept in her spare bedroom, she made everything so delicate, delicious and dreamlike. She had a nice line in poached eggs, for example. Here's how.

She undid the little kitchen window blind and sort of permitted the annoying morning sun in if it knew its business properly – to mind its business! Then she in a beam of unexpected, unheralded healing light cracked two bantam eggs she titled 'googs' into a boiling-hot saucepan and turned the Kooka Stove down to low. 'Go onto low, you.'

Then she quickly poured a jig of white vinegar into the same pot. Then she attended to the thick Tip Top wholemeal bread; generous were her toast slices, unfailingly generous as opposed to expensive cafes of today in Carlton, where all toast is positively skeletal, Biafran toast.

She scurried around like mad to get the Western Star butter uncold and warmed-up by placing a scud of it on the frying pan, then she'd put her reading spectacles on to better study the dissolving of the pure country butter doing its work and deemed spreadable then for me and entirely edible. 'It's coming – like Christmas.'

She fried sliced green apple in the same pan and moved each browning fragment of those Granny Smith apples about in the foaming firmament of the whizzed-up fat so thin. Then she sat me down plop on a cushion for my bottom and skinny I nibbled the lot and must have said, 'Gee whiz, thank you Nan!' several times in a sleepy reverie known only throughout West Preston itself. I loved her and she me.

I sipped grapefruit juice; she personally hacked a big one up and always said of grapefruit as she flicked all the pink pips out, 'You get your money's worth with the grapefruit, I reckon!' She then took a perch herself and we breakfasted in style in 1959.

My father was always at her to obtain her own telephone but she declined, philosophically saying, 'I hate them.' She trotted over nearby Miller Street to use the public telephone and used to place three pennies at a forty-five-degree angle and when she pressed the A button she heard Dad's voice and that was her cue to hit hard the B button to release enough Capitalism to hear her only boy, the only one she loved.

I saw her place three wet telephone directories one on top of the other in a floppy stack high enough for her to tiptoe on and speak into the talk-hole. She would cup her left ear in the windy phone box to ward off the tram noise and truck noise to hear Len and talk to Len.

Her boy Len in distant Reservoir, four long miles off.

Her depression was her other son Stan, who died when he was twenty-six after coming off his motorbike. He died of pneumonia ironically just before penicillin came in. This true tragedy occurred in 1946 just after his only brother Len came home from peacekeeping duties in the Pacific. What is worse than that, I'd like to know. For the only and older brother to turn up in West Preston and find his brother dying in hospital after a motorcycle crash. They were close. They played footy and cricket together and acted the goat together; in the Great Depression years they milked cows at Bunyip in Gippsland because Pop, their dad, got out of Melbourne knowing a dairy farm would feed them. My dad got into his dark bedroom with a world-shattering migraine for days to mourn his brother properly.

It is said that when Stan Dickins died my bereaved dad went into a ten-day coma. He told me one day forty years ago he simply couldn't believe or bear it. He told me in his cups, 'The merest light gave me a splitting headache, so Mum pulled the blinds down and I went out to it for all those black days and nights trying to believe and bear the unbearable truth of his dying like that and leaving me lonely for him.'

Stan was my dad's dearest companion, I mentioned his Christian name just last week when I saw my old dad and his eyes moistened instantly when he heard me utter it. That is love indeed, I'd say.

Gertrude *would* tell the farm stories, and on Sunday nights when mechanically she Houdini'd into our dim kitchen, she spoke so tenderly of the favourite cows, especially Bessie who wore ribbons in her swishy soft mane. Gert tied them there, when she milked her.

A tiny snippet I heard long ago from Gert was the one about a swagman who turned up at the farm near Drouin, looking the worse for wear, and Pop asked him what he wanted, and the swagman said, 'Could I have a halfpenny's worth of cream please?' My grandfather replied, 'Did you bring your scone and jam with you?' My old family used to urinate with mirth at that, die, slap their sides and literally fall about as though it was the funniest story ever told.

Nan and Pop only ran the farm a couple of years, then returned of course to West Preston as a triumph over starvation in 1935 when the Depression was officially deemed over, but naturally various wolves were still at lots of people's front doors and getting in through the back door too.

Pop was a 'spec builder' who constructed lots of Cal Bung residences around Preston, the Cal standing for California and the Bung for, I guess, Bungalow, or maybe it means deafness.

I remember the summertime trips to Sandringham beach when we were growing up: the energy unlimited and laughter untrammelled. It was 100 degrees in the old Fahrenheit scale of stickiness but nothing could stop our buoyant nature. My mother gigglingly throwing a spongey red rubber quoit on a couple of quoit-poles dug into the hard-packed beachsand.

Laughing at the off-handed catching of the quoit and all the energy in the world at her disposal.

My dad the nonchalant natural-born athlete leaping like a stunned porpoise or a sparkling salmon at the net-of-quoits. We took so many games with us to the beach fifty years ago. We were pack mules. Beach umbrellas and snorkels and face masks and comics and novels and fantastic, large, soft and so warm new Dickies beach towels. The compartment on the beach train was crammed with us and our beach stuff.

A fragment of a love memory is my paternal grandmother guarding me against lethal sunburn by putting her body over me. I was five, at Carrum beach in 1954's summer edition of family life, and she realised that I was fast asleep and shielded me from the furious dancing rays that burn and sizzle and can prove fatal for infants. I, blissfully asleep as a little child, snoring in my adenoidal fashion, framed by prance and strut of waves that soothe and protect, she cast her strong but compact frame over one of her grandsons, and received the sun burning of her life in my stead. This is of course sado-masochism, not heroism.

She could hardly get on the train at 'Sandy', as we called Sandringham, she was so red-raw. She could hardly walk due to the intensity of the terrible sunburn. She refused Dad's offer of some sort of gentle ointment he happened to have on him, like some kind of barrier cream let us say, and so heroically sat on the hot train burnt to buggery just grimly staring out the evaporative window at houses that baked like she just had.

She was sick as a dog at her home. We used to catch the train to Reservoir but Dad'd hop off at Thornbury station to accompany his mum to her place then see to her and make sure she was all right and so on, then he'd walk back to Thornbury station and wait in the heat for his one, the Reservoir rattler we used to call it as it shook you apart. I felt so sorry as a little child for my sunburnt grandmother.

She adored me, and I, her. We were the same except she was sixty and I was five. Same big proboscis on her noble face as I developed later on, like a remarkable likeness being developed in a photographer's studio.

In my undamaged memory (to spite ECT) my similarity to my paternal grandmother is stunning. Of all the ones in both clans it is she I loved in a perfect manner, like the dumb and profoundly innocent love an animal feels for someone kind to it. I couldn't wait to sit next to her upon her couch-grass back lawn, her powerful thumbs and tough finger-joints abstractly reefing out the weeds as she spoke to me. She wasn't intellectual but that wasn't what I was after. She wasn't simple but good with words and observations, but like my father not a spontaneous liker-of-others. Indeed she never gave outsiders a chance. They were shit. Over the road from her house lived a prostitute. Nan called her 'missus-over-the-road'.

Unlike her, I loved people I didn't know; they were a tribe somehow, a mixed-up family of man or a brotherhood of unknown spirits to whom I felt overwhelming rapport. It was like a longing or a reunion when a stranger in the street joked with me, even cried with me within seconds of an unplanned meeting. I've fallen in love that way, often, and never regretted it.

But she trusted only the family and the rest could go to the shithouse, not that she swore or even blasphemed. It was her joy to be with me because I was the son of Leonard her only living God, her only boy, her only hope, her only child, her only son. Gertrude and Barry got on like a weatherboard on fire.

A peace existed between us ever since I met her with all her sisters, it seemed a hundred of them. Bessie who wrote aerograms to her from Noble Park in a fine blue biro – usually those ultra-light fourpenny aerograms were mailed overseas because they didn't weigh anything but Bessie posted them from Noble Park to West Preston, a distance of thirty miles which must have seemed a fair way to her. 'By gee, it's a long way.'

Bessie was four-foot-four high with no bottom denture and worshipped vegetables; that was about all she ever spoke about, the extreme importance of vegetables and their scientific relation to bladder or bowel. She also spoke of vitamins in the same hushed way, telling me at the age of ten I couldn't afford to neglect them.

She was careworn and browbeaten by her husband, Uncle Wal, who was brilliant at being asleep or smoking a briar. Wal never worked and left Auntie Bess for dead once for three years while he sailed to England to catch up with English relatives, while lonely Bessie lost her only child at two years of age pretty much all alone. Bess knew about pain.

Bess endured poverty for forty years cooped up in a thatched hut in a small paddock of unslashed grass with a dirty pigeon coop up the back where Wal kept racing birds that won or died or won when they died. Bessie moved in with Gert upon Wal carking it and I can see them in my mind's eye sleeping together in Nan's home in West Preston. They argued all the day then hopped in together to keep warm.

I adored wildly 22 Miller Street, West Preston, my grand-mother's home, which was a bastion of strength against the outside world, a fort against marauding Indian parking officers, a solace of gentle joking where evil couldn't come and snoring was warmly welcomed. The kettle and the ungulped tea. The wholemeal toast and the two-minute egg and a collapsible paper Christmas bell she suspended from a nail above the doorway every single Christmas eve.

At the age of ninety-nine she died and at the burial she lay in the casket stacked on top of what was left of various other decomposing Dickinses and my father muttered an aside to me as my brothers and mother left the grave with its elementary inscription: 'I may as well get in with her.' Not for the first time in my life I found myself bereft of a reply. He looked so bitter when he said that to me.

At Gert's funeral service it was my mother who wept the hardest and bitterest by far. She was inconsolable, in fact I had never observed her in such a calamitous state of loss. I was talking about her amount of weeping to the animator Peter Viska and he said, 'Ah, your mother lost her sparring partner.'

All those years of comfort and peace vanished now and the safe home my Pop built for her is now so altered I don't know it when I motor past its excrescence. The old toolshed Pop smoked in, which had a real moose's head in it, is over. His musty soul and fishing reels are over. It's all over completely. The only holy relic still intact is its simple concrete number or in fact numbers: 22. It is 22 Miller Street – you can still see plainly the two 2s formed by Pop in 1954 when he built the house hanging on the back chimney. The rest is modern.

So you try to understand yourself after nearly six months in a psychiatric institution, where you come from and who influenced you. She did, Gert, who said, 'No one's better than you.' And no one is.

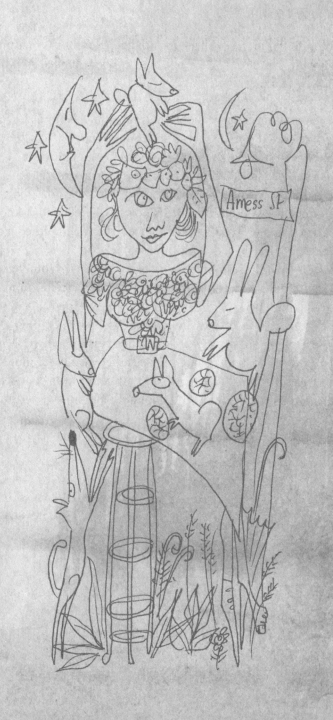

Chapter
two

My mother was born in bohemian Carlton in the oddly named Amess Street, and there among the timeless elms and sunny wrought-iron terraces she was instantly happy, like some kind of human teaspoonful of coffee added to the stunning morning light. She cycled round the dreamy backstreets and kissed moonlit youths without ever tiring. She was very good-looking indeed and adored her father Gus, who claimed he invented stainless steel. He even made their tin sugar scoop.

My mother possessed prettiness and pettiness in that order. She could be shy and charm itself and a brilliant raconteur at the tea table; we never called it a dining table, that was for the rich or at least richer than us. We weren't poor and there were always Weet-Bix on the tea table. We were a passionate lot of pilgrims who loved life in all its splendour and gloom, which seemed to be in the air, in a way omnipotent.

The greater joy in my parents was dancing. My sexy mother loved to jitterbug during the war years and was a good singer and dancer according to her, but according to other reports as well. My father was taught to tap dance and once went into it in the Daylesford band rotunda to my family's awe and embarrassment, mostly awe I suppose. He was quite good in a discounted Fred-Astaire way and the tapping on the concrete floor was deafening but impressive, and we gave Dad a good clap. He bowed. He adored dancing of all persuasions and doted on the Barn Dance and the Gypsy Tap and the Cha Cha Cha and the Mambo and the Foxtrot. He lived for dancing. She did too. They danced their depression off. It was the only way through. Dancing beat it hands down, and they both knew that fact if they knew nothing else. They collided with each other at the Melbourne Town Hall and danced spontaneously like twins. They curtsied and waltzed old-time style and applauded the live orchestra eagerly and ran around the glossy parquetry till late and caught the West Preston tram home, there being no escape.

He was on leave from the war and she drove a baker's cart. She boasted to the family once that her noble steed had memorised the round so perfectly he used to stop outside a residence if Edna forgot whether that place was to have a single white loaf or a double white loaf. Edna groomed the horses in their stable and carried a big, thick, strong cane basket under her right forearm to run the hot bread in. She was strong. She said once the horse stood on her toe and crushed it. She told the agog family the next job after that in the war effort was making parachutes in Plenty Road and then making gussets in a gusset complex; but her stories were always high on the heroic and low on the factual. Like her mother she was a mesmerising anecdotalist, bored stupid with suburbia. They both should have been on the stage.

Another thing about my mother's sheer physical strength I liked was the way she threw herself into washing up the dishes; it should have been the kids' work but we were entirely spoilt. We did the 4 am newspaper rounds but Mum and Dad did everything else. I weeded all Dad's gardens for ten shillings sometimes. Ten shillings was a small fortune in those days.

She scrubbed the enormous, heavy steel roast tray using

Jex steel-wool pads and sang while heaving into the stubborn residual of transparent grey lamb fat. She scraped at the spud tray she roasted them in with the leftover sepia-tipped Jex steel-wool fragments, never missing a bit of the muck left after every skerrick of spud skin was gobbled and thanked God for. She worried at the Gravox gravy pot that she tipped over our Kinglake potatoes. She sighed and sang and whistled and turbined away. 'South of the border, down Mexico way.'

Dad had a bowl of the tennis ball to us kids down the sideway, teaching us the off-break and its best friend the leg-break. Mum had a handful of Bex for a whiz-up. She got addicted to Bex tablets, which contained speed or pseudoephedrine. She adored her brother Henry, who was fearless for a living and as a consequence became a Rat of Tobruk. Henry was the best man at her wedding at Scots Church in Collins Street right at the end of World War II. And then she was escorted to the ugliest suburb on earth: Reservoir, where she promptly contracted unparalleled sorrow.

It was hay fever and loneliness. It was diabolical and unending. It couldn't be edited or understood. The cows in its paddocks were bipolar. Everyone who went there went insane. It was my father's fault they lived in its mud and moroseness because his father built the home in the first instance then gave it as a wedding present to Edna and Len Dickins.

After the war ended in 1945 all you could do of a night was walk to Preston. My parents walked there for something to do, pushing their babies in a pram and possibly weeping. Apart from urinating dogs, there was nothing.

In Plenty Road, Preston, recently all shops were removed. These days the Reservoir-Preston area is a repository for heroin and lukewarm hot-bread shops. In the old days its citizens loathed their jobs and hurried off to their only comfort – the grave.

The clinical depression seeps through its traffic lights like firm

English treacle, making everything black and hopeless. The dirt of Reservoir is volcanic topsoil so that bitter mistrals puff each forlorn flower away. In the year 2008 the only activity on Sunday was to blow your brains out. Or go to the tip and just look at stuff.

My ancient parents still live there in the same small double-brick home my grandfather built in 1945, to coincide with victory over the Japanese. All through the sixties mothers of Reservoir went mad due to the hideousness of where they actually were and how they had to live. It was so barren and bleak you gulped when you turned a corner when you were out walking because you'd only turn into another vile street stuffed full of brick gas chambers.

The frenzied cooped-up terriers of our town's yaps were so high-pitched they gave you tinnitus. Dog fights were popular fifty years ago because they contained real blood, even the hope of murder, but they have gone now, like the steam off a rotten meal.

I wrote poetry in the family bungalow but it was derivative.

I got the old red rattler train to Princes Bridge from Reservoir station which was rather like going to heaven from Auschwitz. I observed the strange ritual of my fellow wage-slaves sort of conversing upon the gloomy platform waiting for the cattle cart but when it shuddered in they got into compartments and completely ignored each other.

So one moment you were chatting about Menzies or the football and the next you shut your fat mouth completely for the half hour the train took to trudge to Princes Bridge. The ferocity of that heavy silence and the paranoia of eye contact only meant one thing. We had no culture. We couldn't be friends. We were depressed.

Often there was even less talk at our family tea table than on the train. We had indigestible jelly and solidified Peters icecream, then my brother Robbo and I played tennis out on the road to cheer up a bit. The ball went down the drain after one hit. It was rigged.

My abiding memory of my own mother is one of unending exuberance and virile superb energy, once called upon always answering in the affirmative. I have this mental Polaroid of her striding like a colossus through our front wrought-iron gate, dressed in a pristine and patterned cotton dress and fashionable buckle shoes, hair exotically brushed and spirit completely gleaming. 'Look out, here I come,' she seemed to be thinking back then.

She is confident and impressive and gorgeously spoken, witty without any fuss or effort. In my memory she strides thus, filled with purpose and brimful of desire: sexual and sensual and virginal and funny. She's got the lot.

Good at tennis and good at the Sunday roast, carving up the succulent lamb called 'a forequarter' that she bought at the butcher's a mile away for fifteen bob, carrying carrots and spuds over the handlebars on the way back home: athletic and fearless and enjoying a chewie and kicking at dogs trying to bite at the meat hung over her handlebars. When she was making a point, she was a good philosopher. A natural-born raconteur.

Whenever my father talked over her in his eagerness to make his point, she mostly let that happen and get upstaged, write off the anecdote, let her heart beat on its own, full of artistic and social frustration. But sometimes she would put her hand up to him, ever so gently, and say quietly to him, aghast, 'I hadn't quite finished, Len.'

And you should have seen the look on his face. Absolutely stricken. Before she got sick, she adored to speak freely and philosophise upon any subject, from the cloud studies by John Constable to the cost of vegies going up, chopping and changing the topics without a second's notice. How I miss her talking to me and entertaining me and joking about this and that in an impromptu way; the same way I speak and write.

It is inimitable.

She seemed like Doctor Jekyll and Mister Serapax. When I was a teenager I used to watch my addicted 45-year-old mother rush to our old family's medicine cabinet and tiptoe up to scramble for the Serapax, an uncounted palmful of them at least. Her drug stash contained several really strong forms of opiates, sedatives and pro-diarrhoea laxatives as well as the fizzy stomach relaxants the poor creature was hooked on. She gargled Eno all the time, even when nothing was wrong with her.

She didn't possess reading spectacles forty-odd years ago so her different-coloured eyeballs could easily focus upon brand names of antidepressants prescribed for her by the GP in a most insouciant way at his desk. My father never did a check to see what was in these powerful relaxing capsules, or whether they should be tapered off or Edna should be weaned off them and live drug-free after six months or a full year on the vile things.

Just as today, the doctors were superior to the workers and honest workers like my father were taught to automatically admire them and revere them. They ought to have been revolted and reviled by them, but in those days it was definitely a 'know-your-place' society.

So my father, tired after nine hours of feeding his thirsty printing machines, used to walk home through Reservoir's only solace, the lanes, and have a decent scrub-up, rinse the muck out of his big blue inquiring eyes and change into his best clothes and accompany his woman to the doctor. I see them now in fact walking together to the doctor's place, arm in arm, murmuring softly, solicitously and tenderly. He knows her body off by heart; he understands her speech perfectly as well as the loss of it through the addiction.

Now it is raining so he places a folded copy of tonight's *Herald* newspaper over her head to ward off the annoying raindrops; they head for reception where six or so timid people sit. They are waiting for their common miracle – another quickly scribbled-out prescription for things to relax you. Valium and Serapax and you are better.

There is nothing of any sort to look at in the doctor's waiting-room so Edna and Len together look very carefully at nothing. After two hours without so much as a cup of tea they are shown in. The doctor writes out a prescription for Valium and Serapax without talking to them, then they go home and she swallows them. Two to feel better, three to go to sleep, five to cook with. She is indifferent to correct dosages and cannot be bothered reading the tiny typeface on the box's edge that warns in two-point type against overdosing. We sit as a nuclear family drugged on a leg of lamb and roast potatoes and minted peas. She makes Gravox stoned.

This was our family's downfall, the obsession with there being something wrong. It's called Munchausen's syndrome. The only thing wrong with my mother was boredom, so she made sure she got her fix. She would have been a lot better off playing tennis or running a hot bath or reading. We stopped having people over and she grew worse and stayed that way forever.

I remember my mother getting ill clearly. She was escorted to the old Larundel Psychiatric Hospital by her girlfriend Lorraine Brochhi, who lived over the road. Lorraine was a volunteer and introduced Edna to very confused patients, one of whom swallowed broken pieces of glass in front of her. Others had epileptic seizures and so on. My mother wasn't prepared for hallucinations like those people. She was so safe and unworldly and really belonged in an annexe of Hollywood, a mythic glitter road out of Reservoir that led to Fred Astaire and Ginger Rogers. Glamour.

She went with me time and again to the local general practitioner, who put her on Serapax so she became an addict from day one. Often she guzzled half a dozen capsules at the kitchen sink with a handful of tap water, not sticking to the prescription at all. She also swallowed Valium as if there were no tomorrow. That's exactly the sense Valium gives you. There isn't.

In short we lost her to drugs. And overdoses of them. Literally bucketfuls of them. Becoming vague as a matter of course. Internalising everything. Remaining indoors on stunning days. Declining any invitations to birthday parties unless they were celebrated at our place. Anxious about nothing and frightened of everything: continually clinically depressed. So many mothers on the tranquillisers and off life.

Distrustful of parties. Gloomy 24/7. Saying no to a dance on the patio. One out of every two homes have overdoses going on in them, drugs that are so incredibly powerful administered by confused siblings. Half the country gulping Serapax. The other half jogging depressed. It's a lethal combination of a foul landscape and prescription antidepressants. Citizenry slurring words like alcoholics but they're not on the bottle. Mumbling instead of coherence. Muttering instead of marvellous. All bent over and picking on their fossilised husbands. And general practitioners in every suburb scribbling out more scripts with those nimble wrists of theirs. It's an epidemic, depression. Doctors have a lot to answer for.

My exhausted father was better off burying the Japanese in the jungles of New Guinea, as he did with a bulldozer in 1944, than trying to comfort a hysterical old woman in 2008. He understood burying the Japanese. They were his country's enemy. But the drugs are beyond his ken. He just gives her more of them and is lonely at ninety.

When my mother was forty she got herself hooked on Bex tablets. They gave her a real whiz-up, especially when she played tennis. A jaw full of Bex all crushed up and dissolved into her central nervous system. Scurrying round after the ball as high as a kite. Laughing oddly. Drugged to buggery. Later at the tea table incapable of sense. Then Serapax and the gas heater on high too.

I lay awake and thought of her lying awake in 1963 when she went through her first nervous breakdown. I saw my sick mother standing nervously by the rockery in our old suburban backyard and she was all curled up yet oddly standing still. She had her old olive-coloured cardie on and the old olive-coloured big buttons, and a bow was in her hair that once was auburn before the anxiousness pulverised the dark brown out of it and the fear hammered the lustre out. She was saying goodbye to my youngest brother Rob and he was just a kid attending school and she was clutching her dewy hands and working up the slippery fingers where she's to savagely nibble the cuticles to their stump.

'Goodbye Rob,' she is saying over and over again and yet she, of course, is going nowhere. When she was forty she had a typewriter and I hoped and prayed she would write down her thoughts, or keep a diary or something, record her whimsies and mysteries, of which there would be trillions because she was once such a good rememberer as well as being amusing, quick, observant. A mimic of the ordinary and mocker of the dreariness.

My mother hated housework. I can remember seeing her bad-temperedly stacking our ugly chromium kitchen chairs on top of the tea table, I think upside-down, the six ugly chairs made of yellow and grey vinyl, and then powerfully giving the cramped kitchen a good going-over of Mortein fly spray. Like millions of honest mums across our continent she stored great faith in brand names, brainwashed by telly, and the words 'Mortein' and 'Fly-Tox' were holy to her.

Half a century ago there were these big, strong, steel pump-cans you could pump insecticide into your family's lungs with and destroy their remaining eyesight and hearing. She violently pumped the shocking stuff into the kitchen with all her might. Cloud after thick cloud with the terrible eye-stinging stuff until she was satisfied or ran out of it. Then with a big chromium door key she locked up the back door that led to the patio and we all had to wait an hour for 'it to have a chance to settle', as she put it. Then she opened the door and we had tea amid those atrocious fumes.

She used to put a dreadful protective muslin cloth, like a vast embroidered fly-proof veil, over the plates and dishes and pre-set knives and forks and spoons, and what have you. This she lifted off with a real flourish and said loudly, 'Sim-Sala-Bim!' as we beheld the various vittles.

The way she served up the fried barbecue chops and rinsed the slugs from the home-grown tomatoes it was glaringly apparent her heart wasn't in the cooking. Like lots of women bored stupid with the vacuousness of suburbia she was really an artist in some way or other; in her spirit she was born artistic and performing the burnt chops wasn't what the doctor ordered. Home isn't the theatre.

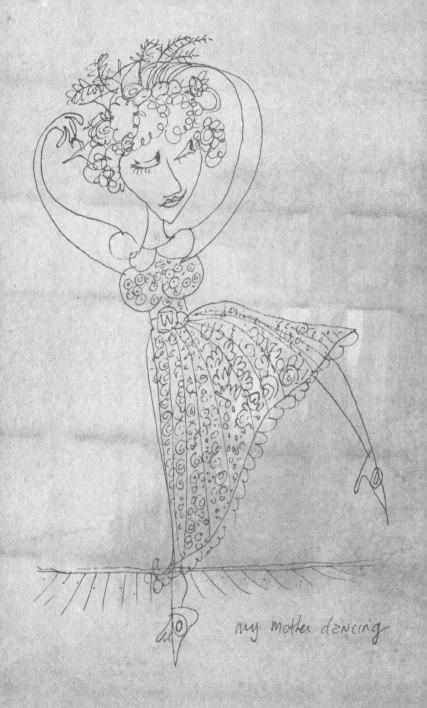

my mother dancing

Chapter
three

IN THE PHOTO album–eyed suburbs my mother and father took their vows and had four sons. I adored my brothers and fought them and forgave them as they forgave me. We played cricket in the street like six million other newborn brothers. Roast lamb on Sundays and indigestion around the television. 'Shut up. *Zorro*'s on.'

It's the immortality you like and the never giving in.

My younger brother Chris nearly dying of bronchitis at the hospital and weighing hardly more than a prayer written on paper by one of us at home. Without being a Christian, I prayed for him in the family bungalow while listening to the first train to work at half past four in the morning. Those were the sounds I grew up with, actually. His breathing and the first train to work. The train was so comforting and melodious because it was the work ethic set to music.

I see as a child of four my tired-out father sitting up late at night at the old pink and grey laminex kitchen table; Mum has gone to sleep in the bedroom and John and I have been read to out in the bungalow, he in the top bunk and me in the bottom one as per usual; we lived and slept that way for years.

My father still smells of greasy printers' ink and although he has stood at the concrete laundry trough for ages scrubbing that ink from his printing factory, he always walks along stinking of work; the pong or staunch, robust tang of the work ethic – you know, never be late for work and never muck up a job. He stood up at big, noisy, heavy, vast printing machines all his life and never was happier. It was when he got home he was stumped.

Now it is night and we ought to be fast asleep, but Chris I can hear coughing in his bedroom next to the bathroom; Mum burns a funny thing called creosote to help him part-breathe and I can remember her lighting it in the dark to get him better, then sitting by him, right by with loving palm.

Dad stares intently at all these intricately tiny, glittery bottles of 1940s photograph-tinters. Many unusual colours – so different from my tiny watercolour box. He has such colours as French ultramarine and cobalt green and Windsor green and pink-lilac and the uncanny vermilion and he bends right over those tiny black and white family photographs he took with his beloved Brownie camera. He painstakingly tints each one with spit and cottonwool.

Down the beach or in the bush he was pretty good with the camera; it was the natural artist and designer in his spirit. I got it from him; he showed me how to paint when I was not much taller than a foot ruler. He intricately dips the razor-sharp point of his terribly expensive Windsor and Newton red sable English watercolour brush, a number '32' made of real camel hair, he said in a hushed undertone; then he squints real hard at John's hair in the black and white beach photo and tints his hair blond but not exaggeratedly or roughly or comically. He's like some jeweller in our kitchen.

Then he tends to the colour green of several types, from deepest to vividest, and all scrunched over the kitchen tea table, his only kind of studio; it is after eleven at night but he is intent and relaxed and all coiled up tinting the Sandringham Beach palm trees green. Then he pats cottonwool over bright and dark spots and frets at the proper blending and fidgets with the pink and introduces cobalt blue to its friend, the summer sky, who is on holidays like all my little family are now.

With a terribly tiny pair of scissors – probably Mum's nail ones – he patiently snips one depicting John sitting happily upon a fence and ends up repositioning my older brother on a watercolour-painted copy of a Walt Disney cartoon-farmyard rustic fence and in the watercolour background my kind and loving parent paints other Disney characters we all know well, like Brer Bear and Brer Fox, and so happy John is tinted in with them, becoming a kind of Disney hero.

Dad had that picture professionally framed and it still sits in proud position near the deep crimson curtains. He loves to tint his family photos and in this new album there are many, not rough, never gaudy, and his best tinting I believe was the way he added lustre and coloured detail on the photograph of my mother's best dress; it is neither a coloured snapshot nor a black and white anymore, but something in between, lovely.

Another photo he altered cleverly was of our first dog, Mulligan, taken in 1947 in our backyard near the tap; it was all bush then, the home town, Reservoir, dusty and ours. Mulligan posed in a bored way near his bone that was – it was said – the hip bone of a horse, and Dad took his snap then when it got developed at the chemists, my dad snipped that particular shot into a bone-shape and patiently glued it in next to more of John playing in rapture at 'Sandy', as he used to call Sandringham. My father had so much fun mucking around with photos; it took the place of the drawing and watercolour painting he was missing out on because he worked like a Trojan.

My good and faithful servants, my parents, suckled at the work ethic; it was the milk, great milk flowing direct from

Capitalism's breast, which never ceases giving forth its creation and simultaneous destruction. My father was a supplicant, a work-slave of time that was never his to possess; he worried if he was a fraction of a millisecond late for work, he cried out, 'No' if the back rubber tyre he pumped up hard to go to the factory was flat. For if that happened and it happened to be somewhat down in pressure, then the real pressure dawned on him that he'd soon be late. If he *was* late he would be docked, or fined a minuscule portion of his wages and that infinitesimal loss of money was disastrous and unthinkable. He was never late for the printing factory in his life, not one day. That determined, strong, little compact frame of his, as compact and tough as optic fibre, stronger than God in a good mood, rode that heavy bike in any weather, storms or heatwaves. He didn't give a stuff; he was never late. He enjoyed the physical challenge of cycling into a hurricane or a rainstorm or a rainbow or hailstones.

It must have taken him an hour and a half each way in the 1950s when he did it; to Clifton Hill from Reservoir is six miles each way. It was light traffic in those days, lots of Holdens and Fords but no road ragers or tailgaters like today when lunatics clog up our choked thoroughfares. He would cycle down the cobblestone alley that led to Millers Printing in Clifton Hill and take off his pants-leggings, the tin clips that men wore on their trouser-cuffs to stop their precious daks getting snagged in the bike chain and chopped to precious pieces.

Dear old porridge got him to and from. Uncle Toby's. Dear old porridge with a foot of brown sugar over it and prunes and a thumbprint of Saxo salt to make it so thick it had to stand up. The life force within Uncle Toby's Oats got Len Dickins up the hardest slope and delivered him to his indifferent employer in one piece; he overtook stalled buses and swerved cars that pulled out from the gutter without any warning. He put on his grey cotton dustcoat and deftly tied the sash round his trim waist.

He switched on a printing press vaster than Rupert Murdoch's empire; he fed it and soothed its voracious appetite till it was knock-off time. He rode the iron-frame bike back home again and leant it up against our bungalow for tomorrow's use.

Like his tireless mother he had energy to burn and eyesight like a wedgetail; he stared unblinking into all the copy he operated on the gigantic presses for Millers Printing and those genius eyeballs in his head had never failed him since he gained his apprenticeship at Melbourne Technical College before World War II cranked up in 1939; he enlisted in 1940 at nineteen and his mother fainted.

My father's lean, taut body taught itself joy through physical work and that work took the form of printing and collating mountains of newly printed invoices and letterheads and business cards and docket books and printed (embossed) envelopes. He was the official artisan of the embossed envelope. He paid a man to invent a strange heating contrivance that when you gave it a flick it heated up very fast and the printing ink rose ever so slightly in height so you could feel and touch its embossed-ness. They were quite tricky to perfect and my dad used to say, 'They are a bit on the fiddly side but customers seem to go for them.'

In fact he was famed throughout Reservoir–Preston for embossed printing, and customers not only highly regarded Dad's special printed envelopes but also put it around how novel they were, so others made a beeline to Wickfield Printing when he later had his own shop at 80B Orrong Avenue. He was never in his life happier than doing the embossing.

The machine cheered him up and drove away the depression that he hated. The hate of depression is rapture of one's love that is work.

If he could have, he would have run to work he loved it so much.

I think it was to get away from my mother and her nervous jitteriness but he adored her and has lain down his life for his sick old wife.

When Len was going full-hammer in the dustcoat, he was always professional and immaculately groomed, with slick, black hair on him combed perfect and face handsome and smelling of Lux Soap all over and shoelaces tied violently in two bows; he never in his sixty years of army and work had a loosely tied shoelace. He is a disciplinarian.

He liked to joke with the customers in the cramped front office of his shop, to tell a funny story and like an actor he would make with the raised eyebrows and dramatic jaw and grim or comic countenances to please his half-hearted clients, make the bastards laugh and then grab their cheque. Mum was a fellow mocker-at-the-right-moment just as Dad was; she quickly realised joking was the essence of Capitalism at its best. You had to crack a joke to get the customer relaxed and happy and his happiness and approval of your funniness resulted in an instant rapport. You posted expensive Christmas cards to strangers you didn't respect but it was expected. My careworn father used to have a coagulated tongue from all the midnight licking of his own special envelopes and Christmas cards he produced at his machines.

I see my father now all these years on, putting on his grey cotton workcoat, the one with a sort of sash-thing that went through cotton hoops round his waist, thin was that waist, and he tied it on, the sash-thing like a rapidly adjusted belt, and quickly combed his then-black hair and almost ran off to work at the printing factory, the one he got going in the garage.

I did not hear him ever yawn or complain, which was called 'going crook', about having to work so hard. 'Not far to go work,' was his morning adlibbed joke about the closeness of his safe garage. Just throw down a cup of tea and confront his big printing machines in there. Give the fluorescent lights a quick flick on their hanging cords and they'd flutter into bright life.

His spartan up-at-five-in-the-morning commencement-to-work routine consisted of boiling up some very hot water, adding a teaspoon or two of a digestive powder entitled Kruschens Salts, watching and hearing its hideous taste whirlpool then dissolve in the 'hot', then downing it.

He then swallowed, without questioning, six dirty, big whale-oil capsules, for 'eternal life'. He then fried up black pudding, which he loved more than life, and sat and got stuck into it on toast.

He looked at his work orders for the day, put his reading spectacles on to study when they were due. He hung the orders on bulldog clips and they swung when there was a draught; there was always one in his shivering garage.

He reached over to switch on the Heidelberg automatic printing machine and it seemed rather to enjoy being switched on so early, for it gurgled deeply as if from the centre of some ocean, and he reached across and spread printing ink upon a large spatula then spread the oily black ink over the big tough rubber rollers and by that time the Heidelberg Automatic had its convulsion and exploded into marvellous life.

He nimbly placed the lead type into its bracket and I stood right by him and marvelled at its insane reverseness (he could always read metal letters in reverse), then the black glossy rubber rollers sailed over the metal words and the printed pages flew out complete and, it seemed to me, shocked, as if the surprise of being printed at five in the morning, in the middle of winter was a bit too much for them.

The invoices, they were mainly invoices, stacked up automatically and automatically quite dry they all were, then an hour later he had printed something like 10,000 brand-new letterheads or usually the invoices, his staple job, the necessary invoices his commercial customers demanded daily, and away he printed, stacked, repeated and never ever got sick or tired or tempted to chuck it in, as resigning was then called, because the printing equalled food. He locked up at six at night. Prompt.

What a great provider and quietly contented machinist he was fifty years ago. He had a second printing machine in the garage. It was called a Platen and it was made in Ohio in 1898 but he had it fixed up and reconditioned and got some mechanic to rejuvenate it. He stood at that Platen and he just purred.

And the Platen was just as pleased for Len to start him up of a morning, for its sound was like, 'Gee, thanks dear Len. I do indeed feel like work today!' So he had both printing machines belting away by six in the morning, he would peacefully hand-feed the American Platen like a contented father hand-feeding his baby.

His highly polished black shoes on with the bows double-bowed: he was never slovenly. He was the epitome of professional out in his freezing car-garage where it was the known and unruffled world of printers ink and reliable tough steel ink-spatulas and flying chalk-dust in tiny transparent puffs of clouds that came out from a mechanical bellows to rapidly dry his orders, then he'd stack them all up.

When I was sleepily getting ready for state school at seven in the wintry morning, yawning, I always washed my sore eyes (I've always had sore eyes, like all poets from staring at life too much). Dad would rush into the kitchen bearing stacks of freshly printed invoices, letterheads, docket-books and flyers and stack them quickly but perfectly in the sitting room to get bone dry. That was the only time my drowsy mother actually saw him, rushing in without explanation in his neat grey cotton dustcoat and tartan woollen shirt on, buttoned up to the epiglottis, buttoned up to stave out the biting cold-snap; and the wolf was never at our door because Dad wouldn't let him.

He never paused from dawn till dark. He was never bent over or tired, not once. It was called 'getting the runs on the board' or making safe wages. His faithful printing customers got their orders delivered as soon as my mother drove them there in the 1962 blue Valiant. She always put on stacks of make-up and a bewitching perfume called Empre-Vue.

'That Empre-Vue one is worth it,' my cheerful father would cry, because it worked. The customers paid up on the spot whenever Mum confronted them with an invoice and winked at them, handing over the first of the cartons of just-finished printing. How could any of them resist such an attractive woman at seven in the morning? They paid on the spot as she sexily chewed Stimorol.

They were a great, perfect team and they knew it and our home was safe. Safe as the indestructible double bricks it was built with; so safe that the grumpy electricians who tried hard to drill through those bricks broke their drills, 'sheared 'em in half they did' – a favourite boast of my father, that one. 'Jesus, my dad made a house to *last*.' My mother's eyes said, 'Ho hum!'

The garage made the money to pay our educations and school socks and school shoes and school shoelaces and other expenses such as life. He flogged his guts out and understood such objects as time passing and death coming and life coming and the latest new baby.

It was a silent world he respected from his five-year apprenticeship at the Royal Melbourne Institute of Technology, where he trained as a machinist; that's what he was studying when he enlisted as an infantryman in 1940 to fight the Japanese.

He fought the all-encroaching cold in the garage the same way. Never give in to it.

He always stood, for he was a little bloke, five foot five and a half in the socks, on a strange (it seemed to me) cut-off pink top of a wooden ugly table-thing that never was explained to me; this still object he trod on to feed the gulping printing presses. It never moved. It was as rock-still as his idea of God. It just stood there and did nothing. That is why you believed in it. It didn't quit on you.

He fed the machines but preferred the American hand-feed Platen, with its indestructible rubber roller, and he smoked in those days, Chesterfield Plain, strong things they were, and my dad smoked in perfect rhythm with the Platen roller as though they were perfect paramours. His big blue eyes were filled with peace as it rolled away the endless orders from his loyal customers. He knew the Platen equalled money. It printed it all the drizzling wintry day long, it ate up hours and tons of orders, such as Dad's greatest feat, commercial-wise, a real coup to print fifty thousand invoice-books and matching letterheads for Ford.

His vertebrae must have pained him after that! He manfully stood there and printed everything in sight for Ford Australia, then he boxed them up himself and as per usual he used great rolls of masking tape to tape up the big boxes of fresh printing for his biggest-ever Ford order.

Pyramids of the bloody stuff, then Mum drove it to Ford in Broadmeadows with the invoice in its Wickfield Printing freshest-ever hand-printed envelope, stickytaped by hand, upon the very top pile. She pulled up at Ford and all dolled-up she smiled sensuously at blokes pushing trolleys and was introduced to Bev in reception, who paid her and gave her a fresh cup of tea and a gingernut biscuit. Ford paid on the spot in those days, and Mum drove the big cash home.

I had a day home from high school once because I distrusted it, Merrilands, and I lay in my portion of our doubledecker and listened to my old man beavering away in the ten-foot-away garage, undoing cans of cold printing ink, persuading the stubborn spatula to add more Collies Ink to his rollers, I could hear all that easily from so close a distance, then he'd put on the radio and listen to the war in Vietnam as he munched a Strasburg and tomato sauce, big, thick, white bread sandwich as he fed the just-as-hungry Platen.

A gut on him like a sink, a steel washing-up-type sink where all the Strasburg and Rosella tomato sauce and margarine evaporated.

He munched away in ecstasy and never a single drop of tomato sauce spoilt an order. He never buggered up a job. He ate like a saint out there but nippily. He sipped his mug of tea out of his favourite china mug, the one he liked was orange with a metallic gleam somehow to it, like an oil slick. I think it was won at the Royal Show. He sipped and never slurped as he trod on that funny, pink-painted, cut-off bit of table top that he loved to stand on to feed his beloved machines because it never wobbled or rocked.

I lay becalmed in the bungalow and at fourteen wondered whatever in the world I would do for a job when I left school? Policeman, poet, fireman, flower-arranger. The Boston Strangler. I had no idea. What would I become? I was failing at high school. Dad was shocked when he looked at my report book.

His big, calloused, inky thumb pointing at my poor mark for Maths, written there by a mathematics teacher who resembled a tipped-over can of Fly-Tox. 'Gee, son, this result isn't very good.' He put on his plastic imitation-tortoiseshell reading spectacles to study the detail in all of my atrocious achievement in Form One, as Year 7 used to be called. He held the little navy blue school report book up to his sore big blue eyes and saw that I'd failed Maths. 'Gee, son. You only got thirty-nine out of a hundred for Maths this year.' I couldn't justify such a foul result and just looked at him in the doorway. His eyes said 'not good enough' at me and I felt guillotined. I had no idea what I wanted to do when I left school, that sorrow called Merrilands High, where I was uneducated insomuch as I was uninspired for four entire years.

He flew back to his printing in the dark and bright garage and I got out of the imaginary sick bed and just like him ate a lazy Strasburg and Rosella tomato sauce white-bread sandwich and rode my bike to school, depressed. I was as flat as my own back tyre.

It's strange that my mother and father were happy when they both worked. In retirement it became pecking orders. Out of indolence, she pecks at him all the time like a put-out chook. He mutters to himself but keeps eyes averted because she's the boss of the wash. There is nothing of any kind to do but go crook and eat greasy, tasteless, expensive Chinese takeaway that robs them of a fair portion of their old-age pension and gives them both extreme heartburn.

In the old days she was the Spartan and loved discipline so passionately and all that it meant, like riding her dark green pushbike to the butcher's and talking animated and sort of flirting with people like Mister Brewer the butcher of Reservoir, who halved a hog right in front of you. I saw him once halve a pig with his trusty bandsaw while flirting with my mum, and a lot of pig's flying fresh gristle almost landed on her but she didn't care much as he was enjoying her flirtatiousness.

'You don't look forty-five, Mister Brewer.' She'd grin at him as he divvied up the pig with its intelligent eyes smiling wide open in stunning death, like he's a pupil at Merrilands, blonde eyelashes and tongue covered in fresh ice hanging out. 'That is very nice of you to say so, Missus Dickins,' replied the jocular slaughterman, wrapping up a nice pig's arse.

'That'll be three shillings to you thanks, Missus Dickins!' sings out erotic Mister Brewer, banging the impressive cash register with his big pink palm that looked like it suffered from muscular dystrophy, although no other component of him did, just that palm that either struck the cash register or sawed up piggywigs all day.

My weary father locks up his lovers, his machines, now and they do deep sighs and lie in state until they vault into rackety life tomorrow morning early. It takes him half an hour to rinse them down and rinse all the rollers that spread the thin black or coloured ink; he is at his physical-fastest, Dad, when he has to speedily rinse the previous colour off the big rollers and ink up the new colour to complete the order. I have never seen a man move quicker. It is hard work to do, but he achieves it instantly in a jiffy; he had a good bloke teach him at 'tech'. I went there too. People love that place in La Trobe Street. It makes sense, not like the invasion of Iraq.

From his beloved bones I got the need to work and play. I loved it when he came home from work and bowled the cricket ball at me down the sideway. We used a wrought-iron gate for a wicket, and at tea-time he turned up in first moonlight in our road and, carting his kitbag full of metal type from his shop, he unsmilingly or smilingly bowled a pretty good leg break to me at the sideway batting-crease.

He rented a shop to print in after long years in the claustrophobic garage; that shop was comfortless and all he did was transfer his tireless tough body from our garage and stand on that pink-painted sawn-off table-stand on its perfectly flat or horizontal surface and feed the starving machines all day, deafened and happy therefore.

He commissioned a signwriter to paint a sign on the front window of his shop, everything of commercial use, including a three-ton guillotine that conjured up the French Revolution in Reservoir; it was so powerful it could easily trim a phone book in half or even a square of three-ply. I enjoyed it when Dad pushed his guillotine button and it had its overwhelming fit and hiccuped into life. That sign said right in the middle of his window in gold gilt the legend that never was LEN DICKINS AND SON – COMMERCIAL PRINTERS. Though he was desirous of one of his sons joining him in the print game, he knew he was always going to be a one-man show. He adored being an isolate. Singular as a tear on your face.

He trusted the grotty kitchen of his sepulchral printery. At home he was fastidious, neat as a pin, loathing dust-motes and detesting filth even if it was transitory; at his shop he was Bohemian and could butter a wholemeal biscuit or two with a just-wiped-clean ink spatula and talk to this dirty big horse that used to look at him in the dunny. That big horse was over eighteen hands high with eyes so deep and dark and bulbous and lazy; I only went in Dad's print shop toilet a few times, so different from the poor but neat one at our home, with the lav-brush in its right spot and lovely new Dawn lavatory paper upon its correct peg and a gorgeous lid to sit on.

But at the shop the dunny was different and burlesque. The sarcastic horse seriously stood in its doorway and looked straight through you as you sat there in limbo reading *TV Week*, its incredibly convex deepest sepia eyes eyeing off you or Dad out there having a read while the phone rang; its stiff tail sort of swishing and the first fingers of morning light stabbing through the slits in the crooked brick mortar in that reposeful toilet.

The Spartan being lazy was a rare feast for my impressionable eyes. Even the horse that was never tethered in the paddock behind Dad's shop might appear surprised that Len had a smoke in the toilet early some days, or just sat on the lid with his head brimming, not with ideas but just sleeping; it is six in the morning and he has run out of toilet paper so uses the 'Green Guide', which clogs the cistern.

When his black bakelite telephone shrilly rings and vibrates with its mechanical urgencies, he leaps from the Heidelberg

Automatic in his dustcoat and jumper under it and answers it in his mellifluous voice with a rictus smile to sound more courteous in his sleep, with all the clattering other machines belting away like obedient steel and grease slaves, the inky rollers like ferocious gargantuan teeth sputtering orders for local companies like K.B. Venetians.

'Wickfield Printing – how can I be of assistance?' was what he crooned into the freezing cold big black phone. Then the palaver, the buttering-up of a new customer and the comical repartee they pretend they don't like but actually demand if you want their orders. He jokes contentedly to win their trust and is soon printing invoice books for Legato Guitars of Edwardes Street, Reservoir.

It is his unstoppable eagerness to please that exhausts him. In Capitalism you must satisfy your customers first and foremost; later come the first cheques from someone you basically can't stand. You just have to piss in their pocket, as we called sucking up to people, to make your wages and keep the hard-earned home.

My mother in her early forties – before commencement of her worries and nervous collapse and her depression and anxiety, which I seemed to inherit as a double-damnation – used to rise alongside Dad and sip her porridge mixed with dependable wheatgerm; she sat next to her man but never read the paper. Just sipped and stared off into forgiving outer space.

She got herself up and dressed in her best stuff and put on the make-up she bought from Coles; she never bought Max Factor or Elizabeth Arden in her life. She produced a morning puff of Empre-Vue that I always bought her for Christmas and put that puff behind her delicate ears to woo customers who were slow payers and it worked. Then she put on her best shoes, called 'clod-hoppers', and went to work with Len by chasing payments.

They were a good team then and the sons never wanted for anything. Schoolbooks and stuff you needed for school always provided on time. She used to cut six lots of Strasburg and tomato sauce sandwiches back then for Len and John and Barry and Chris and Rob and her as well. She always left the big thick-cut Strasburg and tomato sauce sandwiches in their plump new brown paper bags stacked together on top of the fridge first thing before we trooped off to school.

My DNA structure is made up entirely of Stras. That's all we had for all the years we were at school.

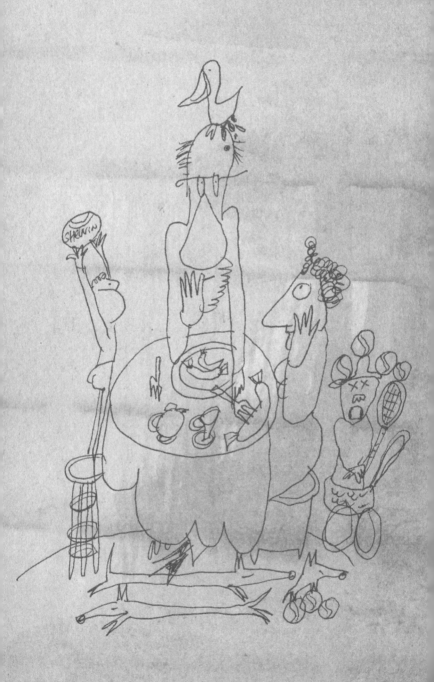

Chapter
four

MY PARENTS ENTERTAINED seldom, being shy, very, but most people in our road were just like them only with bigger or littler noses and hopes the same way. They woke then worked. Then they ate and admired sunsets. The same sunsets.

It was the ridiculously simple routine of daily life that sent my mum crazy; she took Bex, Aspros and Vincent's Powders that she slid pinkly down her teeth mixed with Myra Plum Jam 'to take the taste away', and fled the dreary scene that way with some more fascinating interior view of existence that got flattened out flatter than the pikelets she made on a flour-board made of tough white plastic.

My main memory of the growing-up teenage years is of her baking lots of moist or very dry fruitcakes, depending upon what drugs she was taking and their influence. Her good ones required lots of hard vigour; here's how she did them thirty-five years back.

First she got big bowls out and rinsed them very clean with lots of boiling hot water. Then she dried each with a crisp tea towel until each was gleaming in its way, with a kind of sparkle. She rested the bowls on the stainless steel sink and patted down a few clean pages of *The Herald* newspaper on her limited work-bench. Upon this she set the packets of O-So-Lite Flour.

She patted the O-So-Lite Flour into a whisk object and refined it ever more to rid it of chance granules of imperfection, but there were never maggots. She added fresh milk from several milk bottles and put Western Star butter in. In the end Edna had a good basis for the prototype of the eventual perfection itself; she envisaged it.

She rinsed – although the company that manufactured the delicious Iraqi dates in Tottenham probably had already rinsed them as they got put in packets – great life-giving and death-adoring dates that bore the brunt of eventual family approval in the eating. She mixed the dates into the mixture with a great wooden ladle and plenty of sweat turning up on her honest brow; as she leant over the churning big bowl of it she grunted out, 'You will!' to the stubborn and formless void of still-born fruitcake.

She added citrus peel and glacé cherries John and I used to pinch from their secret hiding spot in a cupboard; they *were* sweet! She put in wheatgerm to give it body, but that didn't taste so great. She tipped walnuts in and dead-set will, but we hated walnuts as they are bitter and sour, but she liked walnuts so in they all obediently tumbled as she bade them.

She got her pretty face now ever closer to the spinning universe of the forming mixture. She included many items with extreme rapidity of intention, no more pussy-footing around. She grunted all through summer for even during blazing summer my mum made fruitcakes before she got sick.

In went honest old Saxo Salt, 'not too much', just a sprinkle or two, then put that to one side as the salt can spoil the sweetness. In went dear old Barnes honey that we as a nuclear family worshipped. In went two big dollops of its far-out golden transparency. After that the glacé limes we looked up to; in they hopped as well because she liked them and used to nibble one. Sultanas from the Sunraysia district and raisins that I could not believe were once grapes on some vine; my brother John, whom I trusted with his opinions, informed me they were made in some sort of vast kiln to dry them all but as I examined the poor sultanas I used to feel sorry for them. I used to imagine their former incarnations, dangling on some sunny vine in Shepparton, with birds whistling as they picked at them.

Now the mixture was right, she put the gas oven on low and patted it all into three big baking trays that she had prepared by virtue of lining each with inside-out greased waxy paper that the Western Star butter came in, in sixteen-ounce blocks. The wonder was the fruitcake dough never stuck to its round metal pot when it got knifed out after it was done. She usually cooked them perfectly, like perfect poems.

The final ingredient is the big brown sugar, big lots. In the end it is ready, sturdy as an Olympic athlete, like some fit, thick-limbed Korean swimmer standing on tiptoe to dive in her oven. She adds now the husky dried unblanched almonds in a circle around the top perimeter of the cake-in-residence and the circle of ballerina almonds takes the cake, as it were.

I am remembering 1963 here, a strange year, one caught between natural exuberance got from dear God and the sickness-addiction of Bex. This reminiscence of fruitcake manufacture is pre-Bex. Her natural high is pure. Pure is best. Best high as in pints of Pura Milk.

She gazes upon the kitchen clock that says in an aside it's time to bake them and not wait round. She never did the pick-up from school; we always walked home and we ran to it to be away from them, the loving parents who slaved their gizzards out. We were spoilt.

Sometimes she spent an extra twelve bob as shillings were called; one shilling was worth twelve pence or the beautiful in-flight bronze kangaroos stamped into their milled mint-new being. What she spent that sum on were diabetes-loving mandarin lollies discovered high atop a packet of mixed citrus peel as a sort of present for buying it. She decorated the top of the fruitcake sometimes, but not every single time, with these sweets to lend the completed cake its miracle. She bent down low to pluck out the genius cake roasted to perfection and let it cool on their own little wire cake-stands.

For decades Mum did the cakes until she caught clinical depression and anxiety. Caught the thing that etches the frown. Got the bug for feeling worse. She gave it to me at birth, perhaps?

Her purpose in respect of the cakes was tennis. She played Ladies Midweek Tennis down at Pine Street Courts in Reservoir each Wednesday morning with a whole lot of other spartan Ednas. They watered the courts which were of en-tout-cas, which is the French for crushed Clifton Hill Bricks; and the en-tout-cas surface was ever so much more pleasant an experience for foot or ankle, as it actually seemed to soothe them as you slid into a hit. The Ednas gave their two courts a thorough soaking during summer, then broomed the tin painted court-lines with a stiff obstinate scruffy brush nailed to a stick so you could really determine exactly where the Dunlop landed and never stoop to cheat. I never saw the Pine Street midweek ladies cheat, not once.

Edna was born in Carlton on the second day of December in 1923, in Amess Street, number 44. She has a younger sister named Marg who is 72 and an older brother, Henry, who died fifteen years ago. She was briefly educated at a Catholic primary school in Carlton somewhere, she forgets where exactly. The only anecdote I have of her primary school days is that a Catholic sister sent her home once because she had her sleeves rolled up and girls shouldn't have bare arms as both of them are wicked.

She cycled round Carlton and loved its fantastic dreamy wide nature strips and parks, I suppose; this is only guessing. She loved her hard-working father, Gus Töll, who was a Jew. He remains an enigma. He once shattered his ill-fitting dentures with a homemade claw-hammer on the slat rooftop of his property. He was up there clonking in a loose slate that had worked loose; his teeth hurt him so he pulverised each plate with a blow. I saw him do it in 1952; I was three.

She took the cakes to the court we played on every Sunday and she also fetched with her in a green bag a hot thermos full of Bushells Tea pre-mixed with sugar and fresh milk, and after a few sets of tennis she sat next to us brothers and undid the fruitcake. The smell was life.

We munched away and it seemed to help in getting the first serve in play. I loved the fat juicy sultanas most of all, and ate into each big slab like a beaver. No wonder I lost all my teeth at nineteen. Dad and Mum versed John and me; or Chris and Rob played whatever combination. We used new Slazenger balls when we were flush, and seconds, they were called, when money was scarce. I have lately turned into a 'Second'. They lose their ability to bounce.

For some reason she used to pick on me more than my brothers. For instance when I was fifteen and still living at her place she came into our bungalow once and I was lazy, possibly growing, feeling luxuriant and enjoying lying in with my limbs taking it easy instead of doing what she wanted, which was to get up. She ran into the snug bungalow and raised her fist to hit me if I didn't get up. 'I'll hit you as big as you are!' she screamed; there was spittle upon her clenched teeth and agonised lips. She mimed me crying out in physical pain and swiped at me and I, in that instant of quickly avoiding her hand, leapt to one side. She frightened me because they had never hit me. 'I'm only growing,' I think I said.

My dad, to hurt me best, cut me out of his conversation; he looked anywhere but me who was in love with him, his words, his body so strong, his feet that rotated as a cricketer and footballer and even a tap-dancer. He once put taps on his shoes, these Fred Astaire clicker things he kept in mothballs in a bedroom drawer, and turned into Fred Astaire on the patio in Reservoir.

My mum and dad never hit each other with any other weapon than silence. The protracted not-talkings-to-you hurt and stayed hurt much better than a clout. They were practising Christians without the bother of church. On Sunday mornings they made contact while my brother John and I attended Bible Class and Sunday School. The Reservoir Baptist Church was an annexe of original depression.

One preposterous song we had to sing at church was to do with Jesus being a fly-fisherman. 'I will make you fishers of men if you only follow me,' it went; at least that is the only line I remember fifty-two years on. I still don't know what it means. Is it symbolism? I thought as a worshipful child it meant tuna or gurnard. I liked gurnard. I liked its name.

As it was her vigour and vital unstoppable health that created joy in our young family, it never occurred to any of us that she could go down. She aerospaced inward and found peace as she soared down right into her bipolar characters, the two Mums. One who should have performed on stage, the vivacity and bon vivant sheer zest, against the melodramatic cry-baby.

Once during 1959 our family got all dressed in our finest to attend a screening of some movie at the new Reservoir Plaza cinema. Dad began well and scrubbed up all the ink off his arms and hands with ammonia hand barrier he trusted to do the job; this was before his own car garage blossomed. He sang in his vibrato and shy way out there with the wash-house door shut fast, the better to croon in an undertone as the ink came off. He and his family humbly nibbled on their rissoles and mashed spud and canned peas, left the dishes for later and went to the movies.

We walked to the corner of Rathcown Road and Cheddar Road then we went up to the line we called the Epping–Princes Bridge railway track. It was a most heavenly romantic-appearing twilight, pink clouds scudding across vacant lots, starry scaffoldings of weatherboard houses being constructed. You had to be there.

Mum looked unreal in her favourite dress, the apricot-coloured one with the belt and golden clasp and a pleasant top with a silver brooch that formed wattle or some kind of yellow buds; she wore high heels to the movie my dad had raved about, some great new western. Not many cars in those days and the motorists had to alight their vintage vehicles to get goats off the main drag, or else they indicated with their whole arm out the window as there were no indicators back then and some cars had a mechanical hand indicating it was braking or stopping soon, and it shot out sometimes when drivers least expected it, but there were never any collisions, not that I saw.

Dad was crossing the road looking good in his best striped navy blue suit and wearing a nice tie tied with the Windsor knot, and his fastidiously brushed black best shoes looked fantastic, and his gold watch wound to the exact right second, but then I saw his mood alter; something agitated him and he hesitated and crossed back over Cheddar Road as if we weren't seeing any western anymore, and that's right, we weren't. He got in a stink. He got in a bad stink over a remark his wife made and to our amazement the film was over now and we had to go home and look at one another again in the tiny cramped kitchen all night. Mum put the kettle on and cried out of frustration. He was a cad! It was boring that night out in the draughty bungalow with bored John and more bored me. For some reason I thought of leaving home after Dad's behaviour. I felt like living in the outback with an Aborigine.

The meal that night after the aborted film experience sank to a *Titanic* low. Dad pecked at his ricocheting peas. Rob was a baby who depth-charged into his nappy while chomping revolting clomps of stewed apple in his high chair commode-thing with a poo pot in it. He ended up with apple in his hair. He's bald now.

Mum sipped a cup of Cottees orange-pineapple iced cordial through a flattened straw and smiled at the aghast clock that always said ten o'clock. Chris wept, then I played cricket with him down the sideway and we ended up playing there for hours in the dependable moonlight. I'd learnt to bowl a wrong 'un.

My strange and unpredictable tribe!

The silence of that terrible night still reverberates in both my faulty ear holes and damaged ear-canals. The not-knowing, the not-having-a-clueing, the invaluable doom that helps one comprehend its spiritual opposite: life! Meagrely putting the chipped dishes in the sink after gnawing on crow, real bird of indignation. Often we ate crow instead of pride.

My father didn't entertain, that was the problem forty-two years ago; he preferred to read in his easy chair with a good volume followed by a wedge of moist fruitcake then profound unconsciousness.

When they managed to have a few friends over it was only Bill and Lorna, whom my brothers and I didn't really know. Mum only knew one kind of party food to prepare for the miraculous moment friends got invited over, and that was Peak Freen wafer biscuits. You undid the things and patted salmon on, then heated them in the griller and gassed your guests. Or canned tuna you could use. Or Swiss cheese or gherkin relish or grated delirium; the options were yours. My parents didn't use liquor so they served iced ginger ale, which makes you giddy after a couple of gallons, but it proved a sound choice and Bill and Lorna guzzled quarts of the stuff as they cha-cha-cha'd.

Politics were never discussed though my dad voted Liberal every election without a qualm; my mother is Labor. She liked Gough.

Dad didn't drive till 1970 when he let Mum buy a brand-new Valiant Charger out of a showroom in Upper Heidelberg Road for $2000. It was quite quick – 65 kph in first gear – and Mum drove without bothering much to stop or give way to oncoming opponents such as biscuit vans, which were just an annoyance. She was scary to drive with.

A snapshot from 1968 I love depicts Rob as a happy and contented little boy with blonde hair and a regal bearing and a great smile and he is standing right by me and I'm on a mini-bike I bought from Ray Burney, who lived a few streets across from our road. The mini-bike had a 50cc petrol motor attached to it and you had to push-start it. In the snap I am on it with our dog Flash, who was a black and white at his chest kelpie-cross, he was such fun to be with. I look so normalised in the photo of the two relaxed brothers, so does Rob, so does the kelpie; he is reclining on the chromium handlebars for John to take the photo of us all. Peering into that old coloured photo a million memories come back reminding my spirit that we had a lot of fun before drugs. Happy were the birthday parties, happy Christmas Days, happy funerals. Happy everything.

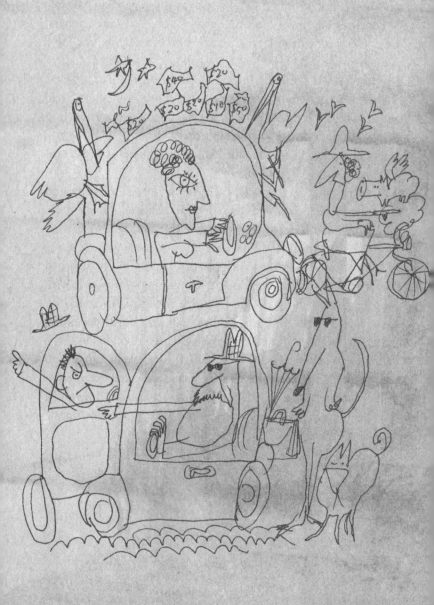

Chapter
five

I WAS SEVENTEEN when I paid off a go-cart in the old motorbike part of Elizabeth Street near La Trobe Street, that corner where in the late 1960s there were many impressive shops that proudly displayed Harley-Davidson and Triumph Bonneville bikes that went like mad. My go-cart had two 150cc petrol-driven rear motors mounted onto a red-sprayed, thin, steel chassis with a racing wheel and groovy, low, thick black rubber tyres and disc brakes. It could go over 140 kilometres per hour no problem.

It didn't have a speedo but I used to overtake motorists going flat chat up Cheddar Road, Reservoir. It ran on BP Zoom and I always checked its tyre pressure as well as its level of oil.

In 1968 we took it to Venus Bay in Gippsland, on Ninety Mile Beach where my father's battalion comrade Mick Lewis had a claustrophobic beach house set in a block of saplings that never bore any leaves. Dad couldn't afford a beach house, he whinged to us, but of course he could; he just didn't want to rock the boat. He was a master stay-at-homer; Dad was a recluse and expected his sons to be anti-social scone-digesters. It was prophetic.

It was beastly at Mick's beach cottage. He was sort of cheerful but used to flirt with my mother in a way she didn't like much, waggling his gingery eyebrows at her and making innuendos. She detested going there, as did I. But the fun was to pack-mule the heavy go-cart over the sand dunes and get it going on the tight-packed sand beachscape and achieve over 140 kilometres per hour with both petrol engines shrieking away.

My brothers and I quite early one morning hoisted the go-cart over our shoulders and carted the cart for ages up winding trails that in a prickly kind of a way finally led to the water. The waves were transparent gold and viridian green. Some desultory kids were flicking Frisbees in a gale and particles of shell went straight in your eyes. We were ready for anything.

I tipped the can of BP Zoom in its lovely scarlet-painted gallon petrol tank and chucked the pourer away and got in it. You had to push-start it so John and Rob and Chris pushed it, then I got out and helped push it down a sort of a slope on the hard-packed sand, then it coughed politely and started up loud. It coughed up black smoke and I got in nimbly and revved it.

It made a sort of whine noise until I really put the foot down, then it screamed full-bore. I murdered a seagull and achieved what I put at 120 kilometres an hour. Ah, to glide smartly across skinny pools of briny sea water and scatter the infernal seagulls, those flying rats.

Rob was young so he had a go with me steering but I let him steer too and he yelled out and had joy and rapture in his innocent eyes all right; although he wept after a few laps because shell grit had got lodged in his eyes and he endeavoured to rinse it out in the ocean but that seldom works in my experience. You really need tap water with shell grit. There was no tap on Beach One. He just had to hack it and use my hankie. John drove the Falcon alongside my go-cart. Going by his speedometer, the go-cart got to 140 kilometres an hour.

It was Chris's go next and he got up to the 140 mark; he wore a crash hat but I'd forgotten in my haste to put one on, typical.

I identify with Toad out of *The Wind in the Willows*. Pretty well thoughtless. John filmed us racing the go-cart with his 16-millimetre movie camera he mounted on his shoulder just like a Hollywood professional as he shot us going full-hammer on the glary bright beach at seven in the morning. I watched a Greek guy eat a raw fish that he'd viciously stabbed. There were Italian peasants out bending over thieving pippies that are protected now; I think they come from the family of clam.

I was nineteen, still sleeping at my parents'; my father came into the bungalow at three in the morning like a summoned ghost. He sat on the below bunk where I always snoozed and almost as though he'd been rehearsing what he had in mind to tell me: 'I had a nightmare about you, maybe I went to bed too early; I don't know why it came except that it did. I dreamt you lived in Carlton as an artist and as a result died in the gutter.' I said, 'Which gutter exactly?' but he didn't laugh. He then went into the kitchen and made a cup of hot Milo.

Seeking the anecdotal origins of my lifelong battle with depression I examine my past fifty-nine years' worth of ecstasy and agony in order to understand some of them, and it's worth it because you then find who and what made you become the character you happen to be. The disastrous and comic elements in your DNA.

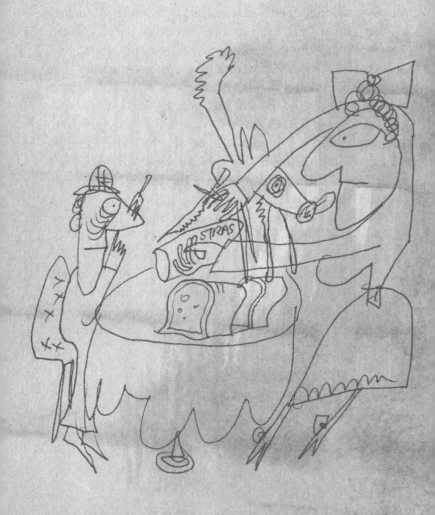

Chapter
six

A MILLION FAMILY REMINISCENCES float back after ECT in my solitary familyless ward. I never had Bex until I was twenty and got a migraine after leaving home and quarrelling with my father, who wanted me to stay there or get married. It was a real pounder, that migraine, as though I were coming apart.

I got a job painting scenery at Channel 7 in South Melbourne. It paid twenty-seven dollars a week less tax but lots of overtime so I was able to put a bit away. I lived in a boarding house in Park Street, South Yarra, that cost me twelve bucks a week including the free use of an iron, except I didn't know how to use it. I still don't.

I had no idea how to look after myself and used to iron my trousers with a big, heavy book that was there. Although I had an oven I didn't know how to ignite any of the jets on it. I dined on a hot pie from the local milk bar every single night for a year, and a tin of canned peaches with a spoon. I used to draw with mapping pens and Indian ink all the time. I got by.

The South Yarra trams made a great deal of fuss rumbling around the bend that led to Domain Road, so much so one couldn't entertain because the chairs shook alarmingly and no one could hear. I enjoyed the sight of tram headlights gliding round my Edwardian antechamber.

I had a girlfriend who was frigid or mad. Or both. Instead of wild passionate sex, which was what I wanted, she gave rehearsed readings from Dale Carnegie's tract *How to Make Friends and Influence People*. I didn't enjoy any of those and was pleased when she was gone with her dopey book. We went to the snow once and she told me off for bending over. She could just make out my hairy arsehole.

I used to walk to work and loved the scenery painting. Everyone was strange at least and I made friends with Gerry Humphrys, who was a musician as well as a psychiatric nurse. He was enjoyable for a living and one day at work he discovered a runover clarinet and just put some gaffer tape over it and played Beethoven perfectly.

I slept at the boarding house and ate Vita-Brits for breakfast for six months or so. I read a book about looking after oneself and that seemed to do a bit of good. I examined a book that depicted the correct way to make your bed and I learnt in the end how to do a hospital tuck. The sheets were folded so violently you cut your throat if you turned over.

The other tenants ate alone in their breadcrumbed rooms and mentally hanged themselves. My girlfriend refused sexual intercourse until marriage. I went for long walks. I conversed with hobos and treasured the wind's monologues. I was a poet in the making.

I brushed my shoes with dark brown Kiwi boot polish and buffed their hides up with a velveteen thing I bought in an op shop for looking presentable. I combed my hair and let it grow. I wanted to look avant-garde. I went to jazz and blues coffee lounges and became an existentialist in Exhibition Street. I read Albert Camus' *The Outsider* and identified with its themes. But nothing ever altered me.

One afternoon I visited a girl I was friends with at a hospital for mental patients. It was out in Kew somewhere and all I did was let her talk about it. That was all she wanted really, to release her demons. It was a good visit because of a kind of exorcism that took place. I suppose I counselled her for she ceased her demented screaming.

I was half an hour late after the lunch break because I couldn't catch a tram and my boss at Channel 7, Ray Watt, the appropriately named Head of Lighting, sacked me as soon as I entered the workshop. There were no second chances, he explained and I showed contempt for the firm. I reluctantly cleaned out my locker and picked up my pay at the pay office and went home to the boarding house for my nightly Four'n' Twenty and big pot of Bushells. The sack was a major blow to my pride, a day off my twenty-first birthday.

It was a dispiriting weekend in South Yarra and I walked the Botanic Gardens to a standstill in my brand new gloom. I fed the unminding ducks and felt envy for the lovers wandering through the Monet waterlily pads. I telephoned my father long distance from Toorak to Reservoir and had to confess to him I'd been sacked. He told me there was always a bed at his place. The long walks, like the walks of Burke and Wills, at least sent me to sleep.

The next Monday I applied for a position as an artist at *The Age* newspaper in Spencer Street and because I had a proper folio I got it. Thirty bucks a week. I tried to look better at *The Age* and lay-byed a nice brown suede jacket with impressive elbow patches on each sleeve to look like a professional artist. I had a nice desk and my first job of artwork was to touch up photographs of dead Australian soldiers. The staff artists were Christian Scientists. A depressed job-lot of them.

I learnt to fry up lamb chops and boil burnt broccoli on the Kooka stove in my boarding house room and that proved better than continuous pie. I planned to be a gentleman and dined with antique silver forks.

My girlfriend was horrible. Wouldn't go the grope.

I had Christmas Day in Reservoir, which is a contradiction in terms. My grandmother made lamb and garlic brown-bread sandwiches and my mother cooked a splendid giant leg of lamb and trays of roasted vegies. We drank an imitation form of champagne called Bodega which murdered your innards. I rinsed my cup of it down with six Panadol.

I sat with the family near the barbecue my dad built with me in 1956 with rocks we found in the Darebin creek, and my mum sang memorably because she was off the drugs at the time, preferring the Bodega. I undid an expensive-looking Christmas card from my girlfriend and sipped my Bodega and Panadol and a hate note fluttered out. It was pure bile.

She accused me of all sorts of things that weren't true and said if we'd had sex she would be cheapened by the sheer physical degradation of such an abominable act. After the party I drove over to her place in Caulfield and saw her screwing her father in the front bedroom with the utmost passion. I drove home to the boarding house and made a mental note to sleep in next day, till five in the afternoon at least.

I appeared to be suffering from some sort of injustice. When Ray Watt sacked me the rot set in. When my girlfriend sent me her hate note my world collapsed. I had about two hundred in the bank and no future.

I studied the Situations Vacant in *The Age*. There was nothing as interesting as what I was doing so I stayed there with the Christian Scientists. My boss was a guy named Ernie Veitch who deliberately developed tufts of oily white hair all over his forehead. One day he gave me a terrific job of caricaturing. I had to draw pictures of famed Australians for a popular book called *Who's Who*. This was in 1970.

I loved that job and executed some nifty cartoons of Billy McMahon, Jack McEwan, Bob Menzies, union martyrs and gargoyles of all kinds. To my sheer stupefaction Ernie Veitch tipped pools of Indian ink all over them when *The Age* editor, Graham Perkin, came in to say howdy. Ernie must have thought Perkin might disapprove of my style or the fact that I was too young for such a job.

A fine how-do-you-do.

I went down to *The Age* canteen and just sat there numb.

Editors munched their revolting salad rolls, which went all down their front. Photographers photographed their own parmigianas. I felt stupid. Disillusioned and shabby on the inside as though my spirit had slipped. Gone down several notches. I ordered a Vegemite and Coon roll and devoured it. A girl in the Art Department called Robin Stewart, who had freckles and a nice smile and wore her hair in a bun at the back, started chatting to me. It was a pick-me-up. She was so sunny.

She told me not to concern myself with Ernie Veitch and the others but to be glad I wasn't in Vietnam where the war was on. That was true and she rallied me. We had rapport. She told me she lived in a hippie commune in Elwood and called the tenants there 'kids'. I was also a kid, she assured me in such a way she made me laugh. I liked Robin Stewart.

One night I couldn't bear the isolation of my boarding house room any longer, the sausages in oceanic fat and the dinging of the trams a foot, it seemed, from my insomniac pillow, and at eight o'clock I caught the Reservoir train and slept on the family couch like a dead ghoul. My mum couldn't wake me in the morning. She thought I was drugged.

She made me a nice breakfast of fried black pudding on Tip Top white-bread toast and ran me up to Reservoir station in the Charger. She used to chew Stimorol and drive flat-chat, Mum did. We listened to rock music for the ten minutes it took to get to the station. Creedence Clearwater Revival. I didn't get to *The Age* until one in the afternoon.

You had to punch a time machine in those days and your timecard got thumped by a black ribbon to show precisely what time you got in. Ernie Veitch docked me a full day's pay but I didn't care anymore about that sort of stuff. He was the Right Wing. Robin told me there was a room available at her home.

The old Edwardian house at 74 Tennyson Street, Elwood, was the antithesis of my box in South Yarra because it had a big, energising, leafy garden and large high-ceilinged rooms with intricately ornate plaster cornices and heavy panelled doors and a big hundred-year-old bath with heavy golden taps on it and marvellous leadlight windows and I was shown a complete bungalow. It was eight dollars fifty per week and had a double bed in it. There were possums fidgeting on the roof and warm old blankets that students had slept in for decades. Poxy ones. Fleabitten ones. God soul ones. My ones now.

It had a little desk and a good chair if you wanted to write a poem on the spot or late at night when the moon was up. I took it.

I didn't have much stuff. A few books and a fountain pen and watercolours and pencils. Robin and I caught the eight o'clock city tram from Brighton Road together then a connecting tram to Spencer Street. It was nice to relax again with someone friendly. She was easy to be with, on the loud tram or in the miserable *Age* building. That night she introduced me to the kids. Like *The Munsters*.

There was a kid named Robbie Rosenberg, who had lustrous black scrolly hair and a jittery giggle, who joked a lot and was pretty serious a lot and went to a psychiatric hospital a lot. It was Royal Park and it was horrible and heavy and kids received ECT there. Shock Therapy. It was called 'Zapped'. It still is.

There was a long dangly street kid called Dave who was friendly as a fireplace. He wore old shapeless grey jumpers and baggy trousers with pockets without change in any of them. He was introspective but also a sort of father-figure and cooked all the morning oats. He had short hair and a lot of patience with some of the nervous ones who behaved strangely, or it seemed that way to me.

At least a dozen kids lived there including a well-built motor mechanic named Rick, who seemed out of place because he barracked for Collingwood and said he loved his father. That wasn't very fashionable. A guy named Barry Batteley was in one big room where he lived with his motorbike. He once sent us a postcard from Darwin addressed to his motorbike and only made sense to his motorbike. He was a scream, that guy.

A thin, acned girl called Toni White used to wear exciting T-shirts with no bra all the time and laughed a great deal on the big sofa in the middle of the carpeted lounge room where the kids gathered to all rave together. She had big inquiring black eyes and great sensitivity and great kindness. There was nothing she wouldn't do for the kids.

I caught a virulent chest bug a fortnight after moving into the bungalow in winter and sweated like anything and shook like a leaf out there so they moved me into the nice big front room for a time where it was warmer. I recall a Greek couple screwed with tremendous commitment the entire evening I had the flu and was running a temperature a trifle higher than normal. They never ceased their furious copulating until midday next day and I staggered out to the communal bathroom and swallowed a half packet of Panadol and crashed for twenty-four hours; I was unavailable for comment. Why didn't they get sore?

Food was scarce at Tennyson Street, indeed it didn't exist; only in our overwrought imaginations were there edibles. We just sat together in the living room starving and tried not to think about fish and chips, puddings and the food our honest parents consumed, like rissoles and mashed potatoes. Gravox. We were lost.

At ten at night, with the rest of the night unendurable, I got up off the floor, where I'd sighed for hours, and walked a mile to the fish and chip shop in Glenhuntly Road and ordered five dollars worth of chips. The guy seemed surprised at such a big order because the usual order was a buck's worth and you got a heap of hot, fat and yummy chips for a buck thirty-eight years ago in Elwood. With complimentary vinegar and thick caked salt. There were drunks hanging around his shop for a sober-up Chiko Roll and some of them looked pretty dangerous and were throwing back alcohol in cans. Steam off the wire basket of chips banged down loud on the butcher paper and vinegar doused everything, even the drunkard's hair. The chips would save the kids' lives as they hadn't eaten for some days. All they'd had was AktaVite mixed with hot water and a soggy Vita Weet.

I grabbed the mountain of volcanic hot fried chips wrapped in so many hot sheets of butcher paper and tissue paper and drowning in vinegar and shoved it under my right arm and ran home with it before the guy could do a single thing about the terrible theft. He said something like, 'Hey, wait on you!' I was deaf to all entreaty.

It was raining mystically and I sprinted the whole mile back home again to 74 Tennyson Street. The starving hysterical kids looked so disapproving when I plonked the great bag down on the floor of the living room, where there wasn't a crumb to eat, not even for a mouse.

I undid the fish and chips like a magician and first of all they looked put out, as if I'd pulled off a terrible crime against humanity. Then they pounced on the chips and devoured them by the fistful or just about wept as they gulped into them dipped in sauce on bits of newspaper. They hadn't eaten for a week. One of the kids called me a hero.

I started to like AktaVite mixed with boiling hot water after that chip feast. Some of the kids had depression and camped in bed all day; such a lethal thing to do at any time. They looked like journeyman ghosts.

As I observed them rip into the thieved fat with such eagerness they looked to me like Oliver Twists without the fiction and I thought there and then of their own parents stuck in a Reservoir like my hometown. Mowing the concrete grass. Eating the same stodge.

The boredom of sameness. That's what creates depression and anxiety.

Some were intellectuals and some were simple but the simple ones often suffered more exquisitely. Tuesday nights became something I dreaded. It was called 'Confrontation Night' by Dave and the idea was that all the kids perched on two dusty cramped couches that confronted each other and you showed no restraint. You let it rip and told one another exactly what you thought of them. It was an extended truth session and polite manners were jettisoned. They whimpered, bleated, entreated, cajoled, swore and blasphemed. Merciless, terribly raw, emotional. A whole lot of screaming going on that lasted five hours until it was AktaVite time again and they went to bed restless and writhed.

Wednesday was Rice Night. I ate my rice in my bungalow sometimes; it got caught in my throat after a lot of introspection and quarrelling.

I re-read Albert Camus' *The Myth of Sisyphus* and played tennis on Sundays with my family, getting away from the freaks to bed with different freaks. I stayed working at *The Age* in the art department which was my security; although the kids at the commune said security is Death. That was a popular motto back then. Meaningless are the mottos.

One night when I came home on Rice Night, I saw Dave as per usual stirring the goddamned special fried muck in his filthy big iron wok and the kids sitting on the filthy lino floor in the kitchen and there were two strange, shadowy men there talking in a rather subdued fashion, so I listened carefully and they were talking about truth and illusion, my favourite topics. We eventually shifted into the enormous lounge onto the two confrontation couches that seemed to be tired of human talk; if those tired couches had ears and tongues they too would be at a loss to discuss the war in Vietnam or feminism in Elwood or any one of a million contemporary issues. The poor couches didn't want to talk or listen anymore to anything.

I forget what we used to wear in the hippie days but at Tennyson Street it was pretty sombre. I had on jeans I never washed and hair the same way and runners, as sandshoes were called, and some sort of jumper for summer and winter that was sort of woolly. Robin Stewart said I had really fine hair and it was tragic I never gave it a comb or a stiff brooming. There was Juicy Fruit chewing gum in it. She spent an hour getting it out one wintry night.

The two men looked utterly brainwashed. They had been. Brainwashed by a Satanic group up in the Dandenongs. Their eyes were wider and more open than ours. They were big and the larger of the two wore a rocker hairdo. His name was Martin Bradshaw. He was a self-styled Messiah of Menace. His companion just sagely nodded and agreed with everything he said and backed him up a hundred per cent physically; possibly they were lovers. The big Bradshaw guy looked like trouble. He reminded me of bullies from the Reservoir Housing Commission flats who bashed kids out of boredom. They came into the cold kitchen together; they did everything together. They stank like polecats together and had a very alarming stillness about them like they were evil. The Bradshaw guy asked if there was a room they could stay in and Robin said there wasn't and then the Bradshaw man sat down crosslegged on the lino floor and instantly so did his silent companion.

The kids talked to them about other crash-pads, as communes were called, where there might be a room available; in 1970 a room in a crash-pad was about six bucks, but both the men sat so still on the floor in a sort of inward and snickering way, just staring into outer space with the cold draught on them, and the big grim one with the snap-frozen rocker haircut just mumbled things aloud like incantations. There was a long talk in the kitchen about Nietzsche and Christ and Freud and good and evil and Bradshaw said he had been taught brainwashing techniques at a white witch's coven in Sassafras. He used to stare for hours straight into a light bulb. We eventually moved into the lounge room and the talk became more heated. Bradshaw dominated it. He quietly raved about obedience to one's conscience and maintaining an inner dialogue with one's immortal spirit. He talked about love being duty, not joy. He was joy's nemesis. He talked about a higher calling and obeying the only voice that mattered. God's.

He talked about how weak our parents were and how confused they were and no matter what he said you couldn't gainsay him as he had mastery and mystery and misery. He memorised all our names and our nicknames in no time and even though Robin had explained to both of them there was no room, both stayed there. They took over the tottering commune.

I kept my bungalow with the possums on the roof at least but the two greasy men moved into Dave's room right at the front of the house and Dave had to share with Robbie Rosenberg, in the room he was always in when he wasn't in Royal Park, where he was a great deal of the time, given shock therapy but it didn't help.

The next Confrontation Night was taken over by the men who were witches in a rainforest with other Melbourne warlocks. Strive as one might one couldn't make one's point. The talk ranged all over the place from the confirmed sighting of Satan in Kallista to the existence of us at the commune at Tennyson Street. Young strained voices were raised and lowered and they controlled the kids without a qualm and sternly mocked them and didn't bother to pay any rent as Robin Stewart pointed out. Bradshaw stared her down like his countenance was made of cast iron. All he said all the time was, 'Are you sure about that, Robin?' or 'You don't have any authority to speculate about that, Dave' or similar put-downs. He had been tutored how to intimidate kids who were one step off suicide anyway, one small scream off hospitalisation.

'Are you telling the truth, David?' 'Are you telling your truth, Barry?' 'Will you be tested out when you face the Lord?' It sounds perfectly ridiculous forty years later but it wasn't then; it was idiotic but unnerving. They never cooked for the rest of us or ever joked, not once, as a joke could maybe bring them undone; I always thought they had a distrust of jokes and as a consequence a distrust of me. I was their one joke.

They were splendid pigs the way they ate with their hands and gobbled the honest special rice Dave cooked determinedly in his wok unless the gas had been cut off. We had a week at Tennyson Street without power as we couldn't make the deadline. In a blackout we were conquered by insanity and cheapened KGB interrogation techniques learnt chapter and verse in Sassafras. No one smiled. They didn't let us.

'What is Robin really thinking, Dave?' all the night long. A guy called Rick was one of the few who had a job and he took on Bradshaw best and came closest to winning a few psychological points – he had studied Freud at his panelbeater's as well as having bounced at a disco so he was unafraid of the big man with the hypnotic, light grey, allseeing eyes and the eerie Mt Rushmore stillness. Bradshaw said, 'You've got a lot of hate inside you, Rick, and you are very paranoid of it.' Rick lost his cool after hours of this torment and challenged Bradshaw to a fight in the front garden but that idea horrified the pacifist commune kids much more than anything, and endless sophistry and chain-contradicting ensued until five next morning when we hit our mattresses with our tongues hanging out and no saliva left nor energy to speak.

I kept touching up war photos at *The Age,* trying to avoid Ernie Veitch and the other sad Christian Scientists who were as much fun as Bradshaw and his silent witness Gary. I did get distracted and the fun started emptying out of me because that duo annihilated any spiritedness; the kids were staying in their beds most of the day – just as I did in 2008 – and stopped thinking in a random or free way because they were defeated. I cursed at Bradshaw one night because he was so demeaning but he just said there was too much confusion and hate in my spirit and I was a practising hypocrite who wouldn't have a clue about flower-power. I was a fascist, according to him.

I challenged him to a fistfight just like Rick did but nothing eventuated and I admit the kids, especially freckled Robin, were appalled that I could be violent. Bradshaw laughed at me, provoked me, and Gary echoed everything the Bradshaw bully ever did, like white devils in tandem.

One night I didn't feel like coming home so I slept in the front seat of an unminding frosty fire truck that was parked in a caryard in Brighton Road, with my coat pulled up high as it could possibly go around my throat and nothing to look at but Brighton Road. Even though it was freezing cold I felt liberated away from Bradshaw and the scary Gary, who in a way was more menacing than his master. Bradshaw was pseudo-intellectual, misquoting Jung, getting Marx wrong, not certain if it was called Days on the Commune or Life on the Dole, a rant of myopic wrongness delivered with a juvenile certainty that wrongfooted the kids and gave them uncertainty in big doses, though they were nervous enough. The two warlocks ruled the roost. They were always there like cancer. You couldn't get away from them no matter what you did. I tried going back home to live with Mum and Dad but that was the past, another suburb. I didn't need to depress my mum and dad.

'Are you sure you're right, Dave?' 'Are you sure you're not frightened, Robin?' Like all bullies through modern history the two slept very soundly, untroubled by absent consciences, while the dozen freaked-out hippies there slept in a troubled way, getting up to urinate because they were so jittery, with good reason as it turned out. Their eyes, the two demons had slit eyes. All burnt-out they were and their faces were demented.

I made firm friends with Bob Harris, the poet from Cranbourne, who hitchhiked in 1970 to the big smoke to turn up to a poetry reading at a terrace in North Melbourne; I met him at 57 Howard Street, where two gentle people put on paid readings and Bob always read persuasively, if forcefully, eyeballing the nice neat audience from the makeshift lectern. He wore an op-shop army jacket both in the street and to bed and had big thick blubbery lips and great warts between his bushy big eyebrows; he looked like a Charles-Laughton pugilist but for poetry. His father had a bushy black moustache and poverty in spades; they lived in an unsewered slum at the rear of an unlit gravel track and Bob, like a monk, devoted every second to his poetry, writing intricate lines in all sorts of ways before he discovered his true style: genius. He was a genius.

He said to me in a deadly earnest way in a cheap coffee joint one night, 'Teach me to rave, man,' for he wanted to be a raconteur as well as an unpublished poet, and I had been out on the street learning to talk for some time now, and loved to speak in an adlibbed and unrushed way, letting my impressions and thoughts come to me direct from life on the street where the most stunning verses come from, and the best pictures, so Bob and I hung around a lot and I lent him five bucks and he lent me five bucks, that sort of arrangement, like brothers we were. 'I dig you, man,' I said to him and we hugged hard.

He moved into the bungalow at Tennyson Street with me; I had no say in it. It was a bit snug with him in it and he had dreadful adenoidal concerns and the bulbous nostrils were always running with a streaming head cold; he was all blocked up and snored something shocking, but I liked him, put up with it as best I could in the cramped bungalow, him on the bed and me on the floor sleeping on a couple of doonas.

Needless to say he took on Bradshaw and Gary as he spied them skulking around together like a pair of rodents. The two couches were pulled in ever closer on Confrontation Night and Bob argued passionately and convincingly and seemed to score one or two points, but the witches won by a landslide every time, ridiculing Bob's born-again Christianity and the fact he was an unpublished poet. That hurt him most and he gave his life to it in the end. He must have been prescient. They sneeringly asked him one night, 'Who's your publisher?' which really hurt him as he had none at that stage.

The kids were pacifists and believed in no possessions, as in the lyrics of John Lennon, and were reacting against the lifestyle of their straight parents; they gave the new men nothing to struggle against; they must have surely laughed at us in their room. They didn't bother to fork over any cash for expenses, always managing to have the pick of everything any good, eating fresh fruit Robin bought at the Victoria Market on Saturday mornings, gutsing into it and spitting apple cores out on the kitchen floor.

Things grew worse and eventually the two devils held us all beneath their contempt. They boasted a kind of majestic stride, a regal walk, and glided round the house like lords, making fun of the kids, with Bob and me arguing to no avail. We shivered in each other's arms in our bed in winter. I used to read to him.

Bob moved into another room when that guy had a crack up and then this nice country girl called Allison moved into the bungalow with me, her on the bed, me on the floor on the dusty, old, dark blue doonas again, wishing I had one of these new-fangled waterbeds I'd been hearing about. I was getting a bad back and it got really bad at *The Age,* doing all the touch-up artwork with such tiny little pens and sable-haired brushes humped over the artwork all day.

Allison contributed to the Confrontation Nights, where truth ruled and kids trembled as all their pretensions and illusions were ruthlessly stripped away by the warlocks who had practised exorcisms in Sassafras and could levitate, it was said, and talk in tongues if they so wished. Allison appeared to venture close to beating them on a slim point concerning life after death, the greatest mystery even in Elwood, and it was great she seemed to win the point and so we all applauded her; that didn't go down well with Martin and Gary.

She said there was only one grief and that was not to be a saint.

Not bad for four in the morning fuelled by watered-down AktaVite.

Allison had a certain grandeur and simplicity and it was life-affirming having a soul like her staying with me out in the cold bungalow. Bob's snoring was like a Harvester starting up; he went back to his father's slum in Cranbourne for a week or so, swearing he'd fix the villain Bradshaw. He invited me to stay at his old man's home and so I went along too, for the fun of it.

It rained determinedly as we walked along forsaken Dandenong Road, rained relentlessly hard and no semi-trailers ever picked us up. We must have walked fifteen miles from Elwood on the left side of the road with our frozen thumbs out and the truckdrivers either swerving to just miss us and give us a spray of rainwater all over us or giving us the rude finger gesture and laughing. 'Our fellow Australians, man!' screamed Bob. 'Aren't they generous! They have bags of room in their warm cabins!' He screamed at them, 'You are the admirers of Franco!'

Eventually we got to his dark old home in the backblocks of redneck Cranbourne where the only things of value were anything you could eat or a car that went and made it to Melbourne. Mud and barking mongrel dogs and thin snags in white Tip Top bread for tea drowned in sauce washed down with bottles of beer and tons of furious smoking.

I got set up in the freezing garage and there was an easel there; that was pretty hard to credit actually, it just seemed so unlikely in a place like that, however there it was, as well as plenty of stiff old paintbrushes and duco and petrol and turps so I started a great big painting of a Christ sort of guy in the manner of Rouault.

I didn't care that it was cold in the Harris garage. I was so sick of juvenile philosophising and tenth-rate profundities and listening to what could only be called rubbish for months on end. I was really sick to death of Confrontation Night. It was sort of enjoyable strolling the paddocks of horrid Cranbourne with Bob but it was exciting to listen to him recite his poetry, even if he was influenced by every poet from the great Dante to Christopher Brennan, our country's first symbolist.

It was so bad at Tennyson Street when we got back, two of the kids were at Royal Park and the place was as low as you could go, with Bradshaw and Gary absolutely controlling everything, and Dave valiantly striving to keep the place a haven for free speech and an oasis for justice, but he wasn't looking too flash; he looked jaundiced to me and was muttering things I myself couldn't follow when I met him again that time.

A new guy named Vin Mangan moved in but didn't stay long because it was so loud with the warlocks; he and Bob moved to a house in Glen Eira Road.

On the most awful night imaginable Bradshaw murdered Allison. He beat her head into the wall repeatedly until she was dead. Melbourne's top criminal lawyer at the time was Frank Galbally and he got Bradshaw off. He said in court that Bradshaw's intentions were altruistic, that what he had done to that girl was on the highest possible grounds, that he wanted to exorcise the devils out of her and was in fact a perfect Christian. Bradshaw got three years. There is no justice. After doing three years, he ran a milk bar in Hobart.

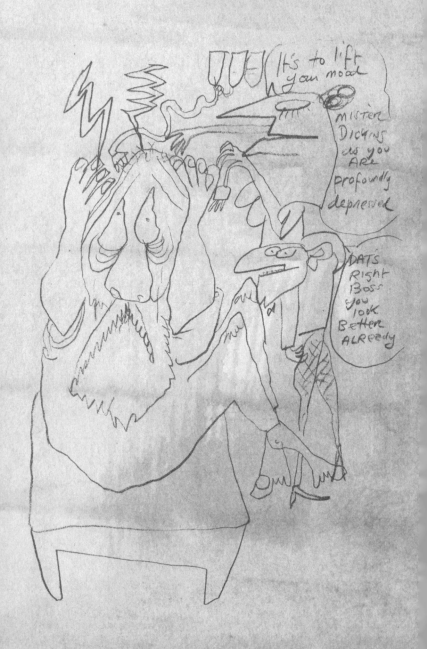

Chapter
seven

I HAD A penfriend, Sue Murray, and she lived with her parents in West Tamar in Tasmania, so I flew over to stay on her parent's dairy farm. I had met her in Sydney, a nurse with infectious humour. The only thing her introspective Anglican father said to me the few days I was there was as he sat on his tractor and tried to start it up. Through his letterbox mouth he said, 'We live in hope but die in despair.'

Staying on the Murray farm was the beginning of my depression, I know that now for certain. We had been passionate in Sydney when I went up there and had made love in a cheap hotel near the Harbour Bridge and laughed, but now she mocked my anxiety and sneered when I spoke of Bradshaw and what he was capable of. She didn't want to read about it or discuss it, even though I'd lived at the murder scene, right *in* the murder scene. 'Get over it,' she mocked. 'So what?'

We quarrelled and I left, not having the vaguest clue where in the world I was. It was an easy hitch to Launceston and I went into Casualty and told Reception I was mad. I couldn't stop thinking of the murder in my home at Tennyson Street. That brutal slayer of her tender spirit. We were all more or less complicit as we should have cast them out on day one. They ought not have stayed there. That should have been *verboten*.

The *Herald* came out at night and it was a much better paper then. The new version, the *Herald Sun*, only really publishes interviews with grapefruits. The *Herald* ran a page-one story on the Bradshaw murder and the Galbally defence, which was more like an acquittal. I remember going up to Dad's place with dear Dave, the nicest guy on the commune, and Dave stood on the patio and discussed the murder with Len. My father asked Dave why they allowed Bradshaw in and Dave said he didn't know the answer to that, then my father said Bradshaw should have got life. 'Three years!' was all he said, incredulous. My mum made Dave a cup of coffee and a tomato and Coon sandwich and we sat in the sunshine near the barbecue. There was nothing anyone could do for Allison except to bury her. It was a violent, brief, shocking news story, that's all, and next day it would be forgotten.

At Launceston General Hospital I was put into the psychiatric wing and given medication I felt was too strong, but psychiatrists always win out. One is too sick to contest the point. I was put in a ward containing bipolar others and trauma others and schizophrenic others and suicidal others and talking-and-gesturing-to-themselves others and vomiting others and endlessly weeping others. I was given a pair of floral shortie pyjamas and a hard bed with a hospital tuck. The nurses were flat out trying to keep up with the demands placed upon them by the mentally unwell. A constant stream of unreasonable demands.

My memory was fried with the stupid face of Bradshaw and the angel face of Allison, my own feelings for her unborn child and my feelings for Allison's absent grieving boyfriend. I couldn't stop reliving it and Bradshaw's face burnt through everything in me. He was in fact traumatising me, haunting me, destroying me.

I was comfortably skinny in those days and kept pacing the slippery corridors sort of chatting to myself, trying to purge myself of the shock of the new murder. How different it felt from murders in films that were artistic somehow, how different it felt because it was real. Although I didn't see the murder I kept re-imagining it, re-imaging it. Bradshaw banging her bloodied head into the wall over and over. Bradshaw pleased with his good work, the work his masters tutored him in, taking demons out of people, getting only three years for it, running a milk bar not long after. Allison and her baby taken out of life by this creature who was beyond understanding.

Each day at Launceston General Hospital I re-examined every aspect of it. Each second it had a re-run in my head. It must have been post-traumatic stress syndrome before I was aware of the term. Bradshaw got the headlines; she got the grave.

I saw my psychiatrist each morning at 8 am. You unburdened yourself then went to the community canteen and had your cereal, which was much more satisfying than listening to the clichés espoused by the superior analysts, the university-educated morons. The dilettantes. Why do you blame yourself? Why do you revisit Tennyson Street? Why do you inwardly scream and outwardly experience paranoia? The questioning was more harrowing than the experience. The psychiatrists in stark white shirts and stark white words and hygienic vowels. Talking about hell as though it were an idea and not a reality. I writhed and wriggled and couldn't lie straight in the uncomfortable bed with the comfortless pillow and graveside manner.

I thought Sue Murray might visit but she didn't. She said I'd flipped out. I'd always been happy in a way and loved lots of things, such as painting with watercolours and pencil and pen and ink drawing. Just being with my family made me happy and contented when they got happy, by singing or dancing on the patio on a birthday party or eating the chook at Christmas.

Now I was conquered and knew it. The distraction was endless and no energy and the body shuffling off to God knows where. Fidgeting and peeling your nails and biting them to their stumps and wondering why I had the luck to experience the shock of a senseless murder. I was beyond interview. I spoke entirely in riddles and answered in non sequiturs. The confidence dashes from you and your thoughts avalanche and you can't bear the catastrophic feelings in your body. Ten per cent of Australians this sick do commit suicide. Will you join the list and leap off the roof? You feel worse and worse and worse until recovery seems farcical, theatrical, unreal as the depression that's got such a grip on you like an iron fist around your throat, your thorax; you swallow and gulp loudly, in fact you cannot stop the gulping.

In short you are afraid.

Some kids there had been interfered with sexually by their pederast parents, which had clearly driven them over the edge into horror that's inexplicable no matter how sympathetic the nurse is. In the middle of the night you discern moonlit outlines of sleeping or insomniac sufferers, some singing out names incoherently, others coherently, others trying very hard to be brave, others wetting themselves.

I circumnavigated all the corridors in 1970 and restlessly strove to overcome the disastrous physical sensations such as shivering and aching and perspiring because the gas heating was up too high and the food made me retch and they wouldn't let me use their telephone because that was a no-no, whereas one genuinely wanted desperately to talk STD to one's parents, just for a second, but it was all a bureaucracy.

After a fortnight of blankness a male nurse came into my ward, sat on my bed and said my form that I filled out when entering their clinic let it be known that my favourite pastime was tennis, so we went out onto a crushed brick court with a pair of racquets and a few fairly good Dunlop balls and even though I was a paranoid wreck and mis-hit the first few exchanges we managed to play several decent sets, the first to six games, and I felt pretty good for a change. I hit a few drop shots and he hit a few good lobs and I felt the lightness return to my legs and the joy was genuine just to run around and get a bit of exercise, not just sit there in the crummy room staring at drugs in bottles and being told it was medication time, even though we'd just had it. Do they want you to be a drug addict? Why are you overdosed?

The birds whistled each to each and we ran around for hours on that court together; in the end I had managed to forget Bradshaw for maybe one hour. My memory was screwing his face into my face like a circus mallet, every second I was seeing him murder my friend Allison, seeing all her gore spattered on the wall, my wall. The friendly nurse took me to a bench in a pleasant green sort of hospital garden and said, 'Unless you improve soon we shall have to administer electroconvulsive shock therapy to lift your mood.' I didn't want it and didn't receive it and he said I ought to sign myself out.

I didn't recognise my signature as I fumblingly signed out, it was so unlike my old familiar one; I who had signed my name a thousand times on drawings couldn't believe that scribble was me. I couldn't hold the biro still and sort of threw it at the discharge sheet. I'd always signed with panache. I thought that was the end of my life, my personal history, my modern way of seeing things and signing things: to lose that was to forget or force your style, that's all you've got in the end.

I had to grip the discharge sheet flat, so flat, with my left arm while signing with my shaking right artist's hand, the hand my artist father gave me. I grabbed my stuff – I didn't have much on me, a pair of jeans and thick socks and my poems in exercise books and pencils and phone numbers and a packet of Steam

Rollers and twenty bucks in assorted small change – and put my thumb out and hitchhiked to Devonport.

I had no luck getting a lift and walked for ages through what looked like mountains but could have been hilly suburbia. I got out into the good old dark. Stars above my head and doused socks below. A nice family picked me up in a modern station wagon. There was an attractive young girl in the back who grinned at me straight away and handed me a chewie and we held hands immediately. The father chatted aimlessly away and the nice mother knitted and told him to watch the road or we'd all die together and not make it to Devonport. I said I didn't want that and they all laughed for some reason but it wasn't that funny. I told them I'd been at the psychiatric hospital and they all shut up.

The girl said I had nice blue eyes and I gave her my home number if she ever got to Reservoir, which I guess was pretty unlikely. We chatted easily a lot and the pleasant mum handed round salad sandwiches. We pulled into carbonised Devonport, which was so dead it had a milk bar that had a big blackboard with OPEN! written on it in an overexcited way, it seemed.

When I had left Launceston General Hospital they injected me with something powerful, a big needle in the backside, and now it was having its strong reaction upon me. I began to hallucinate and shake and crouch on the side of the road and stuff like that, and the alarmed father drove me to the copshop because that was all he could possibly think of doing under the circumstances. I shook like a leaf and fumbled all the stuff out of my bag. I ended up in the police cell as if I were a criminal or something and was really freaking out. My body was flailing around without proper connection to my damaged brain. My mind was finished. I was groaning and trying hard to weep on cue from the sadness of the situation but couldn't respond to sense as I didn't have any to make.

The overhead fluoro cell-light was hurting my eyes with its forked slants, and the cell itself became my hospital ward again in the psychiatric unit. One of the most bizarre aspects of it was that Kath Johnson, my parent's neighbour in Reservoir, was at the police cell too; I mean, what was she doing there? Her nephew was a police officer and she pointed out to me that she was in Tassie visiting him; 'I have always loved you, Mrs Johnson,' I quavered. At that point I wouldn't have been surprised if Captain Ahab stomped into the holding-cell and asked to see my harpoonist's licence.

Two more cops came into the cell and a doctor was sent for, and then my pants were taken down and my underpants slid down and I was gnawing on a handkerchief and my teeth were chattering like a goddamned chimp and I was trying to leap in the air and so on. They shot me up with the antidote to pseudoephedrine, which didn't work for I was still right out of it and raving away like an orang-utan. I really couldn't tell where or what I was. Whether or not I was in suburban Reservoir talking to Kath Johnson, whom I'd always liked, in the friendliest possible manner, or in a Salvador Dali police holding cell in Tasmania.

People were trooping into the police station making nasal complaints about loud noise generated by neighbours or reporting a lost puppy, and the general dreary public-servant work of the cops went on like normal, and there was I, lying under a few blankets shaking and murmuring things that had no intrinsic meaning. The cops were talking to me all the time about where I'd been and how long I'd been in hospital and where I was from and why I was in Devonport, but I couldn't explain anything nor speak of the murderer Bradshaw or his accomplice Gary or mention the commune.

Mrs Johnson kept on saying I'd be all right and soon recover and see my mother but my mother had her own mental problems just like me: she didn't make a word of sense either.

At about six o'clock one of the gentle officers got me washed and dressed as well as possible then drove me to Devonport airport for the bumpy flight over the ocean back to hometown Melbourne. He was gentle; like a loving and protective father, he held my right hand and escorted me to the check-in part of the tiny airport and put my grotty carry bag in where you have to put them in and reached into his pocket for his wallet and bought me a single ticket across Bass Strait and gave me fifty dollars out of his own pocket. All I did was stare dry-mouthed at everything around me and mutter stuff.

'You'll be okay, mate,' he kept on reiterating, 'and soon you'll be with Len and Edna, your loving parents, and you're too young to comprehend what's happened to you and it's not your fault you've experienced a murder even if you didn't see it happen; it has upset you because it really happened in a place where you lived and it's not in a Hollywood movie.' He walked me to the little toy plane and it was raining and storming with lightning all around.

I got on the plane clutching my shrivelled carry bag and drawings. I sat right at the back and stared hard at the airport surrounds and the overhead lightning and listened very acutely to the claps of big thunder and crashes of rumbling air turbulence. I rattled in my seat. We took off on a rough crossing, with the overhead locker doors vibrating unstuck and people's suitcases falling out and the surreal hostesses offering either soft drink or alcohol. The hostesses looked like pipe-cleaners to me or drawings by Dali. The tiny plane really pitched around and some of the passengers looked a trifle put out, as though this pitching-around-thing wasn't the done thing and surely the pilot could do something like turn the storm down or something like that, that's how Western civilisation citizens think. Nothing can stop an Australian guzzling alcohol and so it was that several of the passengers ordered beers or wines in the turbulent crossing, and sipped them as the plane bucked and pirouetted and jerked all around. It was like a psychiatric unit in the sky.

Still the pipe-cleaner wriggly hostesses came bearing nauseous trays of food and drinks. Would Sir like a lemonade? Would Madam enjoy a tea? I was feeling overdosed, and everything in my life, my existence, my history, was catapulting completely. Thousands of impish memories, hundreds of anecdotes and recollections – some not true – bearing down on my young body. I was young then and unworldly.

The plane plummeted down into Tullamarine airport with a screech and a bump but didn't overshoot the runway, as you see in movies of airport disasters. I groggily descended into customs and got cleared to leave but didn't have any cash for a taxi. I recollected the kind policeman purchasing me a ticket home out of his own wallet back at Devonport; indeed he seemed like a manifestation of human kindness. The image of police, as far as ordinary life goes, is cruelty or indifference because they are always fat and eat all the time in cars and couldn't care less about hippies like me.

I hitchhiked up the drizzly freeway and got a ride with a fruit shop guy in a sliding door van with sultana grapes and pears and vegies all in it. He had opera playing on his radio. *La Boheme*.

'Where you going, friend?' he boomed over the roaring of his diesel engine and the reverberating of his tightly packed orange boxes.

'Reservoir,' I answered back in a flat way. 'Jesus, you picked a great night to go there,' he yelled, cupping his mouth with his unsteering hand.

He dropped me in High Street, Preston, and I walked the one and a half miles to my family home, with the storm, so black and inky, never looking like abating, in fact growing more impressive, God really putting on a good show, with flashes of lightning seeming to land on me.

When I entered the old home, the bushes and Dad's plants were bashed by the wind and geraniums had come off, snipped off the bushes by the big blow, and twigs and bits of dusty branches were breaststroking through the air. I rang the front door buzzer and Dad came to the door munching a chicken leg. I must have looked a proper mess to him as he gobbled away on the leg. One of my sons looking like a cave dweller. One of my sons with his unwashed blonde hair on end. One of my sons with his mind missing in action. Shot to pieces by some mysterious sniper I don't know about. I'd better put the chicken leg away and let him in, I think.

I know full well what I must have looked like to him, like a zombie from Tasmania. As if every man who ever goes to Tassie comes home looking like this.

'Mum's got rissoles on,' he said deadpan, the old thespian.

He opened the front door wide and plucked my filthy bag from my weak grip and I shuffled in after him into the cramped suffocating kitchen, the worst room in his house because the fluorescent light on its brass chain hung right down low over your food and the glare was dreadful. My mother smooched me on my unkempt beard and she hugged me hard and said it was good to see me again. My brothers John and Rob and Chris said hi and continued with the yummy rissoles that Mum had added carrot to in the effort to keep the meals succulent.

I had my restless fingers on my cracked lips and fidgeted and couldn't actually speak. I could give zero account of what had happened to me over the past month. It felt the same when we went into the lounge room to have a watch of the television.

The family told me they had followed the Bradshaw case on telly and all of them agreed it was ludicrous he only got three years for murdering a pregnant woman. I sat there mummified by the sarcophagus gas fire and felt vindication just being there with those friendly and so familiar faces. They looked like angels to me, eating rissoles.

I slept in a restless fashion out in the draughty bungalow, with John sort of making me laugh with his innuendoes, but the laugh sound I produced didn't feel like me much. Bradshaw, what he had done, had depressed me profoundly and indeed permanently. I would never ever be the same again.

Over the next weeks I lived at my old home and used to ride my bike around a spot in Keon Park called The Oval, which was where folks played footy and cricket or rode their bikes and so forth, and as I pushed my pedals around and truly enjoyed the physical refreshment of doing so I was trying to purge my damaged memory of Bradshaw. But it was no good. Every word and gesture he created was stamped in my being. He'd de-railed my youth and spoilt my carefreeness. I played rock and folk music in the bungalow and got on the dole at the Preston branch of the CES. The first pay would come through in a fortnight, it was said.

I went back to Tennyson Street to see how the land lay but it was deserted. Toni White still lived there and was standing in the kitchen ironing her floral bellbottom jeans and smoking when I came in. We shared a coffee and she made some stale raisin-bread toast, burnt black on a buckled aluminium fork. The kitchen was filthier than usual and there was spat out dinners all on the lino and rat droppings on the scattered table and a big old concave AktaVite can.

Dave came in looking ten years older and he picked at a morsel of burnt black toast like we did and he made us all a white Nescafé with brown sugar in it and he said it felt good to see me and they had no one in the bungalow and if I felt like it I could rent it again at the same rate of eight bucks fifty per week. I shook hands with dear Dave and moved back in again.

Dave and I shared a burger in Brighton Road the next night and there was some semblance of normality in a cretinous deed like that, and we've always got on, Dave and I. I liked Toni too; she had scored a part-time job in town and so was pretty rapt about that, and Robin Stewart was to move back in so that was uplifting, and they who hadn't moved out after the murder were trying to keep the commune on its thonged feet somehow, but it was over.

Call them flashbacks or post-traumatic stress syndrome or just memory loss or brain impairment but meeting Bradshaw blew my mind. My safe universe was brought undone and my original innocence had been replaced with vacancy. I would be clinically depressed or manic depressed till the day I died, and you just had to deal with it as best you can, mostly by putting up with it.

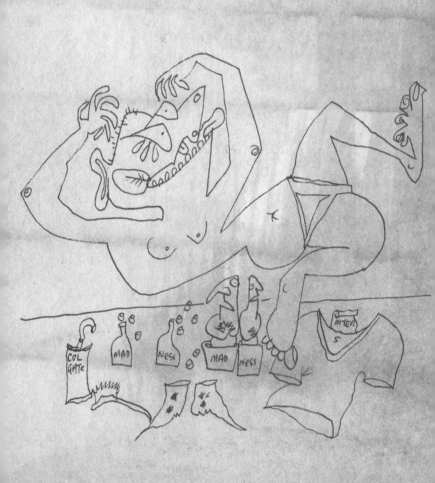

Chapter
eight

DEPRESSION IS NOW like diabetes, an epidemic in Australia. There are so many brutal forces within and without to destroy you. When the marriage breaks down you detest each other asleep. In your comparative dreams there is no empathy nor sympathy for each other's yearnings or sufferings. They don't matter, even the other's health is meaningless. How completely different from when you met entirely by chance and fell in love in 1982; 1982 was my favourite year because I met her in it.

In June, I was flying back to Windsor in Melbourne from San Francisco where I had lived in a crummy hotel that had boozed Negroes lying down at the entrance I had to step on to get to the front door, which had stopped revolving 100 years ago. My girlfriend Rosie was pregnant and had a curette the day after we got to New York even though I argued the moral point to keep it because she might not be able to go to term with her next lover. I paid for the abortion. It cost me $400 Australian, so I had nothing left for the holiday after that. 'Don't you patronise me,' she sneered when I suggested she keep the baby.

The so-called holiday was six weeks of alcoholism and chainsmoking and arguing. I moved into a cheap hotel in San Francisco to flee her. The hotel had fleas. Each night in San

Francisco I dined upon a bizarre form of Chinese soup that had licorice in it. I flew home to Windsor to my flat at 4a/4 Raleigh Street, Windsor: $22 a week with free use of bath. In fact I didn't realise there was a bathtub in it for three months.

My left ear canal exploded on the plane and I've suffered from tinnitus ever since, an incredible ringing doorbell effect. The nurse on that jet told me to catch the bus to Melbourne from Sydney Central rather than fly home, as I could go deaf. I thanked her; and that is exactly what I did. On the bus I didn't have any money so couldn't eat a crumb and just hung on until I got to my flat. My brother Rob was in it, tucking into poached eggs on toast, with hay fever on the side.

As I opened the old flat door to behold him, I observed him sneeze magnificently for ten minutes, exploding watery filth all over himself. He was so red in the face. I had a chest bug so fell asleep in the doorway. He chopped a bit of red gum in the alley and sneezed over everything in sight. There being no bedroom in my old flat I expired on the couch and slept there with my nose to the wall for a straight twenty-four hours; at least Rob said it was twenty-four hours so it must have been.

A few nights later Rob got his own flat in Elwood and left with his hay fever. I was brewing up a soup with chops and vegies. I drank a bottle of claret for my hay fever. My girlfriend Rosie turned up crimson in hue and demanded instant sexual gratification. But I wasn't quite ready for that and continued drinking in my doorway to catch a few lost St Kilda sea breezes. She screamed hysterically and produced a large dagger and mimed thrusting it into her stomach. I couldn't quite take her meaning. She shrieked, 'If you don't come back to me I'll kill myself.' She pirouetted over the fence that separated one slum in Windsor from another. She then made several stabbing actions but nothing eventuated. She then ran hysterically towards busy Punt Road to leap in front of a car. But nothing happened.

Is this her or my depression? Surely the sympathy has to go to her; surely I don't count. But did she intend death by her own hand? As for the running towards furious Punt Road, was that theatre? Maybe she did mean both things but to me it was blackmail. You remember anecdotes like this one after ECT is introduced into your body. She's happy now with her partner – that's all that matters.

My style of prose was taught to me by a stoned hippie up in Sassafras in 1969, when I was a freedom-seeker. I realised I didn't fit in with the conventional persons of modern society and listened most obediently to him by a creek. He was tall and thin and very wise. Robert Fencham – he sat in an op-shop white singlet by this friendly gargling creek and explained that 'the only way to write memorably is to type from left to right and never fuss about punctuation. Grammar is for reactionaries.' I've not forgotten his advice and still type as instructed by Robert forty years ago. It is called 'automatic' writing; there is no censure and no hesitancy between the creative mind and the typing finger or sometimes fingers. It is for me the only way to work and enjoy the process.

English teachers at high schools I've taught poetry and prose at look at me with astonishment or incredulity when I tell them pleasure is the only key to writing. If you feel great you write that way too.

Possessing an elephantine memory during ECT is a charming thing; no matter how determinedly they fool around with my mind they can't destroy it because of that sage hippie in Sassafras half a century ago; he taught me the most valuable thing in life: if you're happy you've got your enemies stuffed.

I caught the bug to drink alcohol at twenty-one and drank pots of beer with anyone I met. Women drank white wine and men beer, oceans of it. After detesting the venomous bite it made on my jaded palette I began reluctantly to adore it, whatever it is it seems to cure life or loneliness. But alcohol *is* loneliness.

I grew up in the drinking culture. You drank or were considered a bore if you did not imbibe. 'Are you on the wagon, mate?' was the common insult. 'No, but I have to pick up my son at his school so just a Coke, thanks.' But they sneered and anyway Coke gives you high blood pressure and who wants that?

Sometimes after a poetry reading when I was newly betrothed I used to come home with a wrapped-up-with-cellophane bottle of red for giving a spirited rendition from one of my books, and I'd grill up some Coon and tomato on toast and enjoy a midnight feast in the sitting room, read something fascinating I'd written myself and get drunk. I'd be assured of a bad night's sleep after that.

I met my once and future wife in June of 1982 at my salubrious apartment at Windsor, where Mr Diemond of Diemond Real Estate drew up the first draft of a one-year lease agreement of $22 per week. In it, I had a TV and me.

Sarah Mogridge was like me, only pretty. She wore her black hair mysteriously over her bright, hazel eyes: the most exquisite eyes I've yet been graced to peer into inquisitively. Her job was to conduct an interview, called a Vox-Pop, for ABC radio. She wanted to understand why as a man I'd done nothing lately but write monodramas for women. I had no idea but after her brilliant cross-examination I began to see why. It was her beauty. She was quick as a goldfinch and a voracious reader of books I'd never get through. She'd read the complete classics from Enid Blyton to Les Murray. Like my father, she could easily quote from all her sources.

We were an odd couple, I suppose. To begin with, we rented cottages together in order to look after ourselves properly and she continued to do that over twenty-seven years together. She won lots of prizes at the ABC for radio production and twice the Prix Italia radio prize in New York. She'd lived in New York and I always believed that it was that city's speed and sophistication that formed her sparkling repartee and instant rapport with anyone she bumped into, including possibly me. We definitely had a regard and sympathy for each other's stage characters and personas. She was a theatre company.

We travelled to Swansea in Wales after our marriage where she sent me up for bursting into tears at Dylan Thomas's place of birth. I went to Swansea from Reservoir as a homage to the man who made me write. I knelt down to inspect the sculptures-into-a-rockery, 'The Hunchback in the Park', in a beautiful little Welsh waterfallen park opposite *his* home and was muttering the lines I knew so well when Sarah pointed gravely to a tap and said solemnly, 'Look, *his* tap!'

She's theatrical and incredible as a person. In 1995, our son Louis was born, my godsend. He's just like her, easily hurt and can't bear a word of criticism, which makes life hard indeed as that's about all you ever get.

In the end my wife's mother, Margaret, approved of me, although I always think her best dialogue spoken live was after the first dinner I put on for her and her third husband, Leonard Legge, at my cramped but suddenly chic flat in Windsor. I roasted gently a baby leg of spring lamb, carefully inserting minute cloves of garlic in it, rubbing a little olive oil and salt on it just as I'd seen The Galloping Gourmet do on television. His name was Graeme Kerr as I remember, and he had a marvellous way of preparing exquisite food in a completely intoxicated sort of way, with various ingredients and rare herbs spilling everywhere. I did as I was bid.

I got to and picked up bachelor filth. Like yellowing copies of *The Age* and the *Sun News Pictorial* and various folded sheets of unimaginable meaninglessness. I didn't have a vacuum cleaner, blast it, so I just acted like an elephant and using my trunk I sucked up anything I saw that an old couple may slip upon, such as useless scripts and telephone directories that didn't seem to make sense. I put up my best collected prints nice and level on their backing-sheet hooks and half-inch nails and saw to the Gravox and rinsed hard my Dutch willow-pattern gravy boat, that boat sunk without a trace; it was the last relic really of anything delicate in the flat to regard in any lasting sort of a way. I peeled the real peas.

I obtained the best vintages and rinsed the best unfractured wine glasses, six. I set the table using my best and only silverwear, had from Kinglake Trash and Treasure. I tipped percolated coffee straight down my elaborate throat. I made sure I was funny.

I put on a nice clean top and tried to iron my pants with a book, which had worked once before. I combed my dark hair (oh God, I do wish it was dark again!) and they knocked right on seven on a Sunday to meet her new boyfriend.

She kissed me on the cheek and we laughed just seeing each other, as it is in the first flush of romance, then her mother cocked her eye in judgement (stern was that first judgement of me) and Leonard awkwardly shook my proffered right hand in an unmasculine (thank God!) way and they entered my hovel. Margaret took off her coat and handed it to me as though I were an usher at the opera; I placed it cautiously over the fridge in the tiny kitchen, where I shot a rapid glance at the food but naught was burnt and I stirred the peas that I'd paid so much for at the St Kilda fruit shop. I lit a smoke but left it under the tap thinking maybe Margaret and Leonard didn't approve of smoking. They smoked like mad, both of them.

They looked a trifle cramped but it was okay, I thought; and Sarah poured us all a delicious glass of cold Rosemount chardonnay to relax with, then we chatted as though we'd always known each other. I put on some music but it was switched off immediately.

Margaret was funny, as was Len, and I thought I'd just met a duo of senior theatricals. They were like characters in my stage plays; I thought they were fantastic raconteurs.

This was June 1982 after my return flight from New York, where on that peaceful journey I burst my left ear drum and it hoarsely crooned to my overcooked cerebrum ever since. About ten at night I presented dessert, which was moist chocolate sponge I'd bought in Acland Street. They said in tandem that they absolutely adored it and I was praised for its unexpected inclusion in the menu.

The lamb was complimented for being charm itself as was the mint sauce in the willow-pattern gravy boat. I rolled a joint using some liquid hashish I bought from an Italian who worked at Johnny's Green Room in Carlton; he was the guy you paid to play Kelly pool on their magnificent pool tables. He wore a greasy rocker haircut and a vile black leather apron round his ample stomach. That apron stashed the hash.

I dextrously assembled the joint. I was always bad at rolling cigarette papers but because it was everything to me, that first-meeting night, to make a good impression I made the joint nice and long and dry and thin. I think I put a ribbon round it. They had a toke. Margaret said it was superb and so did Leonard, who didn't inhale. Sarah liked it and I only inhaled half a toke and made Turkish coffee which I set at their left as is proper in the best circles. I opened the window and let the rain in. Some fresh air was desperately required as it was all a bit of a strain if the truth be told, and I love telling some of the truth.

Margaret told me she wanted to come and see my new play at the Playbox Theatre, it was called *A Couple of Broken Hearts*, and had to do with eccentric people in Yass, New South Wales.

I was stoned when I wrote it and it was a hit with similar audiences. Margaret ended up seeing it but was too sick, I think, to enjoy its weirdness. She had a bad heart. I remember her looking restive before the curtain went up, standing there in discomfort with Boyd, her son.

About midnight the Penfolds port was consumed within six little port glasses I'd been given for a library reading. When I was being silly, Margaret reached across me and whispered to Sarah, 'Oh, darling. You can do better than this!' I was inwardly shattered, then said nothing because I have perfect manners, and saw them down the old concrete stairs to what Margaret called 'their motor', meaning car. She was pretentious but charming in her way, and now she is gone I think of her with dedication and affection. Margaret Ryan always saw to it there were no silences during their meals. You couldn't internalise. You were expected to contribute and talk fascinatedly constantly. Not so easy.

This is twenty-seven years ago. Everything is. I feel twenty-seven years ago.

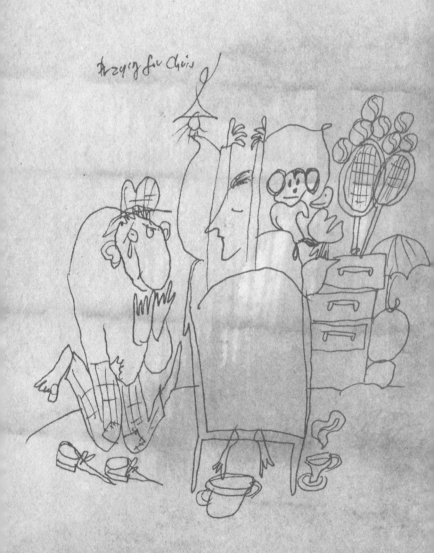

Chapter
nine

WHEN A MAN splits up with his wife of nearly thirty years how do they possibly become friends? It seems impossible for a man of my generation. Do you celebrate birthday parties from different addresses? Do you dress the Christmas tree from different houses? I know I'll get better at it as time goes awkwardly by. I know I'm impossible to put up with. But we were a duet for so long. She is much funnier than me or her elaborate mother, who was like an emphysemic stand-up. Cocking that orb-eye at me like George Formby.

Your young child sleeps in both houses and awakens in different rooms with entirely different feelings in each of them. Being good friends as well as sudden strangers: I mean, how does that mixture feel for your child? It has to be slightly ambiguous, wouldn't you say, for them at thirteen years? He beheld us as firm friends when he was born and when he was her idea. All her ideas come to brilliant life, like a painting.

I snipped the umbilical cord, crying hard, like a trillion grateful happy old fathers, with shaking fingers and through a waterfall of cascading tears of gratitude that he was born alive and happy.

'Don't wait all day,' says the midwife Wally Donaldson, hands on hips. I couldn't see where I was to shear it, shear her from him, give him breath of his happy own. 'There you are,' she said, 'Louis!' She was going to call him George, which I like also, but we likened him to Louis the Sun God, for such he was to us.

The best feeling was taking the newborn babe home in a car that drove properly, pulling all the nut-brown window blinds down to cast out the knife-in-the-eye summer sun operating like a fiend at forty-two degrees all day; the savage slants of sun 'like swords', she used to say, kept out by the cotton blinds, things of sense.

How well I remember my wife, when she was so heavy with the pregnancy, standing by the bedroom window squinting at the early morning damnation of another fiery hot day, and saying, 'Is that fucking blue I see again.' And she never swore. Not much. She's a very intelligent and hypersensitive person who has devoured more books than I will ever get through. She's read the classics from ear to ear.

Laying the contented baby in our double bed and keeping him cool during hare-brained March of ten days consecutively over forty degrees. He gargled icy water in his milk bottle and seemed to laugh by way of baby language. He's either placid or chuckling at life.

She confessed to me years ago she was never happier than when she sat and breastfed him in the comfortable floral pattern armchair in the front room, in the comfy pre-dawn dark before the unforgiving sun came up causing mayhem and such fear. She used to work as a program producer at the ABC and now was at home with the baby, intending to freelance; and I was writing columns for the *Herald Sun* and *Australasian Post* and *The Melbourne Times*, as well as working on theatre plays and novels and so on, you name it, anything written I did it immediately. I was like my father Len, only happy when of use. That meant working on something.

Crisp the memory of the baby crying instantly he received his booster needle at the old Essendon Town Hall, where I took him at eighteen months. All the other babies cried simultaneously in that dusty old hall. From their prams and pushers and in their mothers' arms: 'Have that, little chap!' laughed the needle-gentleman.

Where is that defining moment of physical and spiritual realisation that your marriage has had it? Maybe mine died fifteen years ago when we forfeited our beach house due to my tax debt? I owed $60,000 to the ATO and selling our lovely beach cottage at Venus Bay was my Waterloo. I didn't listen to my accountant and stuffed up big time, too careless by far.

She put so much time and love into the restoration of that quaint weatherboard home by the ocean, and I blew it. It was previously a weatherboard home that lived at North Clayton and some speculator sawed it perfectly in half and rejoined it in a paddock at Venus Bay, where the air was sweet and the trendies hadn't wrecked the place yet. It was still virginal and innocent with free sand bars. Having to sell her dream holiday house must have killed her will to love me. Even fifteen years ago there was a property slump and it was hard to court any buyer. Eventually it sold and I paid my tax bill off with our dream. Marriage was never the same again.

We were so laid back down there and enjoyed eating relaxed instead of bolting it down. We took our time and played a great deal of tennis on the court that was really just an extension of the road through town with a net on it. We had time to examine bush birds and observe their nesting rituals, not that any of them taught me anything about my rituals.

We had a fight one night at the beach home, which to me seemed to come out of thin air, but obviously her anger had been simmering. My brother Chris and his first wife Robyn were staying with us, and it all exploded when I asked her to turn down the music and stop drinking because I needed to sleep. Sarah didn't stop screaming at me till seven in the morning. I cried the whole time she screamed into my body until she was spent. I was the bully but to me she was that. Whenever she screamed at me she accused me of bullying her but it was I who felt browbeaten. We're all bullies.

Chris said they had to be off and started up their car to drive back to Ballarat, but I told him the fight was hot air and to join us for breakfast as she was by now sitting on my knee, kissing me and the hate had gone like a snuffed candle. But he was put out by the crudeness of the all-night brawl and lit out.

My wife gardened at Venus Bay; in fact she loved planting saplings and seeing them come up healthily, well, not quite so effortlessly, I suppose. My job was to 'show no initiative' – she laughed as she said that one – and just tip the wet mulch in or push the wheelbarrow. I loved going to the Venus Bay tip; maybe those trips were prophetic? Heaven is only temporary.

On Saturday morning I used to trot off to Safeway in Collingwood real early to shop for big fresh black flavoursome mushrooms, fresh garlic, butter, wholegrain fresh bread and fresh oranges to hand squeeze to concoct a refreshing breakfast for the little three of us, but now I just don't care. I used to cook chicken fresh and make an intriguing garden salad out of baby tomatoes, spring onions, all that, and toss it and present. It enraptured me to make them satiated and munch well, eat well, chew in harmony and not go the bother of leaving our home and getting freaked by parking officers that book you while you chew mushrooms elsewhere. That used to give me major indigestion!

The end of my marriage has made me not bitter but apathetic about things like cooking. My son's a galloping gourmet and finds many faults in my burnt sausages these days. I'm a rotten chef, let's face it.

I once loved to see my tired wife take a long soak in the tub, it was amusing the way she turned the hot back on with one or other of her luxuriant toes; God knows that with me as the erratic breadwinner there was never much luxury about. I never earned more than $40,000 a year in my life except for the year I worked for Telstra. Teaching poem-creation in schools earns me $225 per day after tax and I cut my own sandwiches and fetch my own Nescafé and sugar and a tiny flask of milk. I offer the children the chance to believe in their own poems and cartoon-drawings; at my best the work is not imitative but pure peace. I'm an old happy hippie.

My favourite school was Ruyton Anglican Girls' School in Kew. The principal Miss Gillies had a pair of silky terrier puppies in each breast pocket and gave them each a twirl over those skinny shoulders whenever she came into reception to greet me at seven in the morning. 'And how is my delicious Mr Dickins?' Then she kissed me tenderly on each flushed cheek.

She adored poetry and me in that order. I felt the same way about her, though she was seventy. She was the only school principal I'd worked for who was light-hearted. In years of teaching poetry in Victorian schools as a resident, she alone was interesting and new each day. She would misquote from Walt Whitman and I could misquote from Wilfred Owen and she would eagerly interrupt me and complete the lines Owen wrote in 1918 that are still a marvel to me. 'My scrumptious Wilfred Owen!'

I taught the kids there how to exploit half-rhymes in the manner of the late Wilfred Owen; the kids were only eleven years old and some wrote elegantly, of course, and loved to read aloud, clapping their palms when the moment was either dramatic or divertingly amusing. Sixteen pairs of highly expensive silver teeth-braces going up and down to the delightful assonance of poor Owen indeed!

Miss Gillies rostered me on to the timetable and I taught all day like a standard English teacher, which I'm qualified to do as I obtained my Diploma of Education in 1974 at the old State College in Grattan Street, Carlton. I still have it in my desk-drawer, the original; I treasure the thing, actually, even though I nearly failed. But it allows me to be the guest teacher in schools and as a consequence it's priceless to me.

Some of the English coordinators for whom I've worked seem distrusters of poetry rather than worshippers. What is upsetting is when one teaches (or encourages is more accurate, really) a very original and intelligent pupil whose mind and writing are superb, but the parents are material savants and prefer Porsches to poetry, and the pair of them, whatever their background and race, wouldn't dream of reading any poem aloud. They also wouldn't dream of reading their child's (or teenager's, more likely) poem that they wrote, using panache, in their buckled exercise book or hidden somehow in a desktop computer. Poetry in Australia is a oxymoron.

I taught poetry at Scotch College (another anomaly – how could that occur?) and the head of English shoved me in their atrium. It was just frightful up there in the eyrie. The sunshine needed to be turned right down, and I had a painful back and it hurt me to sit on a dopey cubist black backless sponge-thing like a burnt pastie and encourage poetry from paint, my only associate. There was a squad of ten boys all elite, who wrote well lying upon their lithe stomachs and scribbled lazily or fastidiously with blunt or sharpened HB lead pencils so I could easily hear their leads spiralling straight through their notepaper. I asked one of them to sit up nice and straight and he swore at me.

One of them was of Indian descent or ascent or whatever it is, shatteringly handsome he was, in fact the best looking young guy I've ever looked upon. He was the equal of Omar

Sharif when he was young, and was eloquent with a voice that was mellow as honey. When he shared, the others listened grimly because he was a standout. He was talented and so were they, but he was so original and gifted with grace as well as intellect; and he was nice. His name was Ben and he wrote fantastic imaginative theatre dialogue, which he also acted out amusingly like a natural mime.

A few months after that engagement, I was reading the newspaper on a certain Sunday in our courtyard enjoying a coffee while my wife enjoyed her morning long shower, when I focused in on a photograph of a dead Indian schoolboy and I muttered, 'That's Ben.' He had died on a bushwalking expedition after his morning tea of walnut cake, and the portions of nuts killed his body. They shoved the adrenalin syringes in him but he was gone. Six hundred Scotch College mourners filled the ensuing newspapers and with all their pomp and dignity I could only think that he was clever and original and undead to me with my recollections of his writing.

God decides the jig is up. We have no say. I often assume my jig is up and the eccentric way I live I suppose is anathema to others-than-me. But I recovered from a clinical depression I suffered for six months by writing and drawing, my only two gifts. They are not jokes but presents from friendly old God, who in His or Her wisdom decided not to murder me, at least not yet.

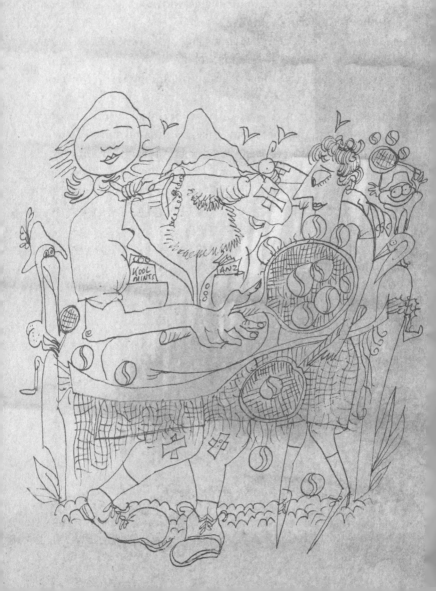

Chapter
ten

MY FONDEST RECOLLECTION of Louis going to Christchurch Grammar School was the time my wife assumed he was old enough to go there by tram. He was in Grade 3 at the time and the walk to the tram stop was only up Barkly Street anyway, a cinch.

She flew off to teach and I manufactured her cheese and tomato sandwiches, popped them in their plastic snaplock envelopes – my eyes watered trying to nut out how on earth to do the seals on them – then I added a slice of her favourite chocolate roly-poly spongecake.

I accompanied our child to the oppressively designed tram stop opposite Melbourne University and checked his school backpack for his Nutella sandwiches and tangerine and apple (he won't eat an apple if it possesses a dint or crude repulsive parental thumb-print, and fair enough). He checked he had his bottle of diluted Ribena with its hard-to-come-to-grips-with screw top in its correct place in its unfathomable bag. He checked to see that he had his new Pokémon collection of beautiful swapcards in their right spot. And his pencil case and his new runners, but he was a bit absent-minded and realised he had them on by looking down upon them, with their laces tied in extravagant bows. He was over-excited to have the chance to be liberated and travel by tram on his 'self' as he put it, 'I like to do things myself, Daddy.' I kissed his blonde hair billowing in the Swanston Street breeze; it was cold and then I walked back home and drove the beat-up white Corolla down ferocious Punt Road from Carlton to South Yarra, like Ben Hur in the hair-raising chariot race scene, racing trendies instead of chariots.

I manoeuvred the car well and got all the crucial green lights on that hazardous road, the main artery from our home to his school in Toorak Road, then I surreptitiously parked where he couldn't see Daddy and actually hid behind an enormous thicket of waving bamboo in the courtyard of a block of flats, waiting to see Pinocchio go by chomping his shiny red apple and carting his schoolbooks. He then did; he looked just like Pinocchio in the Disney full-length movie on his innocent way to school. So innocent, eager and trusting. Since he was born thirteen years ago I have had a good rapport with him; there has not been an argument with unfair existence. I am forty-six years older than my daily tennis opponent.

Like me he inherited a love of any ball that is capable of life. He used to kick a toy football in the nearby park and be transported by the magic of things that bounce. The flight of the ball in the park astonished his sensibilities. He ran after the tennis ball and chuckled at the unpredictability of its ricochets and blurriness and soft focus then he'd catch it as if catching onto the greatest secret in life. To play. If he doesn't play then life loses all meaning.

The astonished park and the beloved flight of the magic ball he learnt to catch all meaning from and to escape from all meanness.

The way, as an infant, he raced after the spinning football was as if the ball were beyond reality or belief, this odd bladder that charmed, intrigued, amused, captured and freed him. At the age of two he could kneel or crouch to put spin on the ball. To put bias on the ball, to give its permitter a twist then explore the way it went to one side slightly or span the other way, the origins of playing cricket older in the friendly park with gigantic elms and swaying oaks 165 years old, so the old people said in their cups.

Before we moved to Carlton we bought a place in Flemington, 63 Illawarra Road. I used to cross the road with him and guide his limbs towards this derelict brick 1920s power station, an ugly prospect for playing, but we used to clobber an old worn-out offshore tennis ball onto its rusted corrugated iron sheets of a roof, and he laughed at the returning ball's dramatic and unpredictable reappearance. The fun we had! It was cheap and silly but he adored it, like a tom-tom drum it kept on beating in my noggin: 'Children *must* play.' The roof was theatrical and the bounding about in the almost-dark did me good, good for the breathing, as dying smokers say.

At Carlton there's a park in Murchison Street where Louis and I played for ten years. On a scooter his lithe perpendicular physique got down low, as low as possible, and steered it two inches from the concrete and winding footpaths. The leaves dwindling and the curious possums at times licking the condensation off discarded Coke cans at approaching twilight. Nothing could stop us playing together; nothing, not even death and we'll not do that.

Even on blistering summer Saturday mornings when all the trendies were out like zombies shopping at IKEA, we played tennis on the curly road. It was difficult to maintain your balance but good for its unexpectedness. We kept that ball in play no matter what. The odd old happy father and the chaste boy with the eagle eye inherited from his Grandfather Len who never missed a catch at cricket, not once.

About thirty years ago when I met my wife, out of fun we hit an old brown tennis ball for over an hour in the centre of

Raleigh Street, Windsor, where I rented, and that was just for kicks, really. We did it out of being a bit shy; motorists tooted us to laugh and point and ridicule something meaningless like playing when you were thirty at least, but we felt like escape.

When Lou was about six we played a funny new game after school called kickball, whose rules were to keep the tennis ball in play no matter what, so you started by booting it into a brick wall. It would then fly rapidly into the slippery dark steel latch of a gate then rebound at a rapid rate into a toilet emission stinkpole or strike the dusty smashed-up window or hit your chest or whatever it did in its liberated way.

You laughed at the random echoes the ball manufactured as it seemed to do whatever it felt like, the ball was the moment and you knew the ball well, me old, him six and laughing and animatedly rushing after its latest angle, hopping over an old lady's wrought-iron gate; youth must be served a ball that lives on its Indian Rubber wits. It was as if the ball was a comedian and it was an actor at the top of its form.

There were rules we made up for kickball but they had nothing to do with scoring points or the dumbness of being best; we were both best. The fun we invented was to follow the mythical Peter Pan concept and give in to him.

I took him to the raucous MCG to follow Richmond, his side, and I was young again in the innocence of his company. I felt redeemed again being next to someone who had never hurt anything. My life as a writer was or is a bitter feud with finance. Never having it easy and feeling the jolt of jealousy especially at Christmas time when Santa urinates upon the have-nots.

An inner and practising Socialist conscience informs me all the time to be mindful of the fate of others. I am always pulling up short in whatever street or thoroughfare I'm walking on and see a man or a woman in such a parlous condition. Impoverished with the struggle of having nothing. I think to myself as I see someone in woe trying to get up the slippery uneven warped concrete steps of a post office, or trying just to cross the road with no idea what they're doing, being vacant, drunk or drugged or dopey from anonymity gone on too long, everything agonising, particularly the fact that no one kisses them forever, and I observe their plight and realise I am different and spared.

Louis ennobles me, lifts my flagging hide and it is only when we two are kicking the football or adlibbing that existence has more than meaning; it has communion. He cheers me just by coming into the space I'm in. The loneliness wisps away like buoyant tea steam. I'm redeemed.

When we still had the beach house at Venus Bay I loved to hold him by his tiny limbs and skim him across the foamy little breakers that formed like the instant giggling he turned into at his sheer delight in the prancing, funny, transparent, cobalt green slapping waves, which he must have seen as not a bad reason to be alive. I skimmed him and the trail of splashes and glee went hand in hand five feet out from the sand.

When he turned up with his mother to visit me in the clinic his noble expression was unjudging. He forgave me for being clinically depressed. He forgave me for being old and confused and going mad from worry over my imaginary family and uncertain future. He spoke to me after I'd had ECT exactly the same way he spoke to me on the street carrying a cricket bat.

He is a blue-blood. An aristocrat.

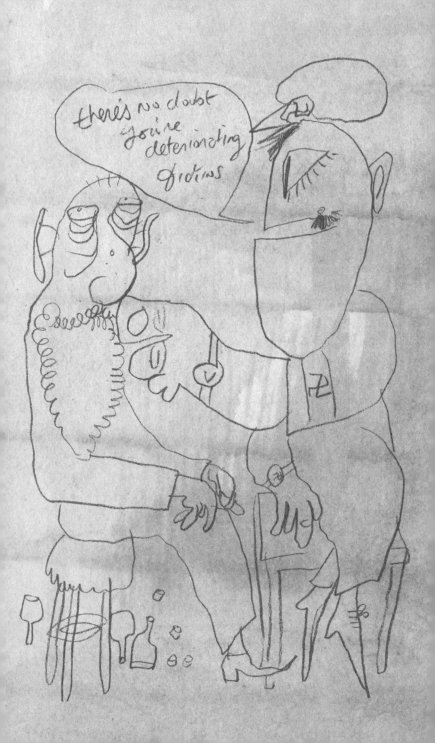

Chapter
eleven

My ERRATIC, light and heavy drinking contributed to the breakdown of my marriage. I can't hold it and don't want it, so I've stopped. The not-minding it is the end of marriage and the beginning of disorder. To begin not to love within the marriage is a miniature harm, or personal fascism where the necessary niceties vanish, to be replaced with frowns and withdrawal. Eating or sleeping separately as we both did – rotten. The result is the breakdown of trust.

You are overweight and repulse her. Fair enough – time to leave. You're better off without me, I think.

When I was a child the fragrance of alcohol bit me and I saw it as liquid ruin. Then I grew up in the drinking culture in Carlton when it was seen as de rigueur to stagger home blind drunk. Amazing I can still draw. My actor colleagues drank during the day and studied the lines of their manuscripts sometimes stoned. You were an outcast if you sipped a glass of milk. You were nothing but a bore if you preferred soda to chardonnay. Milk is nicer than chardonnay any old day in the week. I get drunk on Liptons. I'm a two-bag man.

It used to amuse me to observe my fellow inebriates chuck back ten-ounce glasses of Carlton Draught at a rapid rate all day at Stewarts Hotel in Elgin Street in order to 'get the effect', as they put it. The 'effect' was purple in throat and nape of neck. From reasonably intelligent to stupid in no time, just a whirl of beer taps and beer thumbs and thumbs-up then incoherence. From neatly attired to a bag of shit in the long-benumbed course of a muggy summer afternoon, with blowflies in your flat ale and giddiness for a bad counter-lunch. Dining with indolence and the need of a taxi to bear you home to die. How is this cutting-edge and character-forming?

Plonking greasy champagne empties out at six in the morning. Grabbing at fried chicken amidst galleons of burping empty wine bottles and a disgusting banquet of banalities. Drinking too much is now recommended. After a play I wrote, you celebrated with alcohol and the pressure to be a big drinker was real. If you sipped soda you were an ingrate.

Same thing after a successful art gallery launch. You managed to sell a few new pictures so the crowd pack a restaurant to celebrate the tiny success. The boisterous ones order the drinks and you clink to your kidney failure. You perform a near-perfect impression of Lazarus and rise again from the dead; you had them laughing, all right – that was what they were after – you were the dead life. Something has to go and it is your kidneys and your liver that pack up.

Panadol time at two in the morning but you have a child who requires you to have a steady hand, not just to draw with but to hit the tennis ball, pump up his new inflatable dinghy and undo his chocolate Big M packet without spoiling it or spilling any of it. In short, you need to be straight to be a good father.

I would go off the drink for a month or two and sip vintage mineral water. It killed me to be the decent chap and drink mineral water while pouring my wife a decent white at dinner. She needed it to cope with having to look at her husband, a fat fool.

Then the ecstasy would kick in, which consisted of reading to my son at night in his safe room a billion miles from my drinking mates or me drinking alone in the spinning courtyard, twice a week, considering planets and my own personal cosmos of claret and endless cigarettes.

To be sober and read well to him late at night was the cure for my drinking habit to help beat the pain of realisation I wasn't loved.

To hear him chuckle a lot, that beautiful laugh he produces so readily, to look unbloodshot into his strong gaze, the identical, forever cobalt blue of my father's or my own eyes, was to feel new again. I am after that, by the way, as I write this book on depression. Redemption is sobriety, luckily or unluckily.

The trouble with water, though, is that it just doesn't cut it. You'll end up a cyclist if you don't watch it, and I don't like them. They get in my way. They accuse me of destroying the ozone layer with my 1990 white Corolla sedan.

The trouble with sobriety is envy and I got envious of her enjoying a nightly white or two when I struggled over bubbling mineral waters at restaurants or home. It makes me urinate almost immediately, mineral water; it should be banned at once for the real threat it is to family sustainability.

One night after I got in from a hot night of tennis with a friend, she really gave it to me. She closed the front bedroom door so our child couldn't hear the yelling, and she listed ten faults I'd made in our marriage, one by one. She cited the faults as on a list or litany of sins, using her own fingers to count them off. She'd been rehearsing my ruin.

The angry voice rose higher than inflation. The sinning father was inadequate in so many departments including deportment. She loathed even my beard that so sickened her but it was only there to keep me warm not to injure sensibilities. She used to cut it shorter herself, insisting it looked shaggy, and that belittled me because it is only hair. I only developed a beard to hide a weak chin. She has always loved the spirit of bohemianism and is bohemian in herself, but that is only when it suits. The loathing of a bushy unkempt beard, and the Samson and Delilah trimming of it, conquered my idea of myself and humbled the whiskery self to a point of obliteration where you begin to wonder if you can speak.

At war is the desperation to keep up with the other conservatives in society and put your child through school and pay the car registration and energy accounts, juxtaposed with the powerful anarchist self in the wife who is liberated but stays a devout Catholic schoolteacher to keep the terrace and lose the husband. One feels like an irrelevance.

A long time ago when we were happy and everything was optimistic and love on tap, and we cared for each other so much we used to be hurt, as if struck by a hard palm over the face, if the other missed out on some trifling treat; we lay in the bed and used to nightly read to each other from favourite writing. We'd get up and make a cup of tea for the other and so on. It seems long ago and is.

She prepared excellent banquets for our closest friends and we shopped for items to please them all, fresh ginger and fresh garlic for the salad dressing. Fresh lamb for the roast and our best antique china and her best inherited silverware so the friends of long standing would eat deliciously and speak that way too, with my wife storytelling and amusing them all without the slightest fuss.

Whatever in the world happened to bonhomie? The roaring voices and crescendo of laughter and kids crying needing to be put in a taxi or put down. The lateness was the irrelevancy. The new bottle was the need. The parties never ended and the vows of love that rang in your ears like Geiger counters.

Hundreds of raconteurs and hundreds of chompings. The

delicious and the dead dining together to spite life. Everyone glowing like some human candle and everyone still fresh and everything chaotic, story-creating tension and boredom in the instantaneous gratification of the need to joke and be dramatic.

At the ancient age of fifty-eight I imitated my mother perfectly. I did nothing but lie in bed and watch my little boy go to school through my bedroom windowpane. My wife cut his lunch and she got ripped off paying a buck apiece for his daily big banana at the stinking milk bar over the road to insert in his plastic lunchbox. She spread his Vegemite sandwiches with margarine and hope. I didn't contribute. I didn't work. I didn't care.

I didn't write for the first time since I left high school in 1965. I stopped drawing. I got better at nothing and did nothing all the nothing time. I turned into Edna's Doctor Jekyll.

Do we perfectly copy our parents' illnesses? Their willingness to get ill at the drop of a Serapax? I, who was ever critical of my mother's addiction to doing nothing all day, copied it and perfected my flatness. You've got to feed it. I was the exact age my mother was at when she gave up. She took up clinical depression as some take up knitting.

My hard-working wife cut our son's lunches and insisted on him taking a shower during winter before putting on his school clothes, something he really didn't want to do, and pour him his Coco Pops and run him to high school before he turned up late.

I would hear them both choof off to their schools together and head through the rain or the fog to live correctly by the board, the great board of education and reason. Sick, I would do nothing and just lie there in the upstairs bed and stare at the ceiling in a state of lunacy; desperately trying to remember fragments of my life.

Bits and comical pieces, the rubbish of the past, reciting to myself aloud in the depression-chamber: the poems by Dylan Thomas I'd read as a boy in my father's bungalow in Reservoir. Dylan had helped me by writing the best poems in the English language. When I came back from the Launceston General Hospital after my collapse in the early seventies it was Dylan Thomas's poetry that saved me from the concept of life being meaningless.

The phone might ring and I'd ignore its persistent ringing. It might be a school offering me teaching. I didn't pick it up. I waited for it to be later. I didn't eat anything or drink anything. I didn't do anything. I was so ill. From April 2008 to November, when I got better by myself. I shocked myself back to health. I didn't need therapy.

The first real impact of anxiety came when I was walking with my child up Barkly Street. Because it was ever so lightly raining, I feared for him and put considerable pressure on him to stay at home that day, this saddened him because he loves high school, and I had a fear of being alone all day, and he said to me, 'You're right. I'd better stay home today. You telephone Miss Reynolds.' But in the end I drove him to school. I knew I was anxious and he was just a happy little thirteen-year-old boy who had no right to miss out on things like high school or seeing his friends in his class. It was like being killed by some sort of powerful force of anxiety. I've never been sicker than that day.

Who can tell you how to be loving? Who can lend you the rare book because it's out of stock? Whenever you marry you are in love with happiness, the constant companion, and it's not an imagining nor is it a cliché. We were happy in hundred degree heat.

Going to Paris together after we married in December 1985, I felt weird on the 160-year-old elevator of the Eiffel Tower and we laughed at the sudden ascension and the velocity of the descent. Visiting the studio of Rodin the only day it wasn't overcast, there was a tiny patch of blue that day over his charming rapid watercolours and effortless drawings. We were sweethearts then. Like the living happy boy baby coming through in 1995 when her gracefulness made him that same way.

What you'll not do for each other, when the weariness and wariness are just a joke and you have energy on tap. When you adore not to speak but lie beneath a shady tree as if it's something out of a child's original poem. Wasting time together is so profound, and education or discipline is so meaningless it's just a waste of effort. In our fifties, we needed carelessness again so badly. Money wrecked it, needing it more than the necessary carelessness. Effort is the exact opposite of love then. Sitting in a cinema contented like children, never sighing, when lovemaking isn't avoided and there are no bitter jokes against your body.

You do the return journey from shock therapy remembering your wedding day. The joy and ecstasy of your best friends so happy for you, all gathered together, giggling in the hilarious backyard. Frank Hardy trying to sell copies of *Power Without Glory* to my wedding guests that day in Richmond. My mother arranging my brother John to hurl them over the fence.

Hanging out in Saudi Arabia together. Passing out together. Tending to me when I was sick with a flu bug and running a temperature of some astonishing level; she was my nurse that day propping me up in our son's room with three glacial new pillows and a jug of iced water for my parched throat and bugged-out eyes. Her speedy mind so unpredictable possibly to herself as well as me; so amusing and spontaneous she could have been a stand-up. *Is* a stand-up.

Her morality was realised when she sent freshly trimmed

flowers to the nurse she liked after my release from the clinic. She's a perfectionist and moralist as well as a standout stand-up. It was like living with Lucille Ball.

But I stayed lonely there and so did she, buoyed, I thought, by our boy, but it was too great a burden to load up on his young unworldly shoulders. I should have moved out and lived alone. I was too weak for that decision and so made the wrong one, to stay. I outstayed my welcome like so many unhappy husbands. I hope that she finds love. Someone.

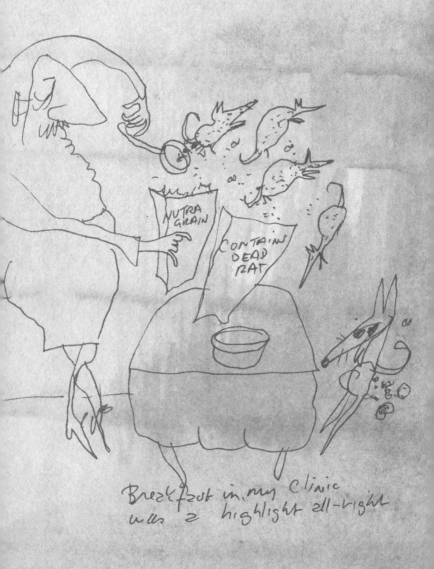

Breakfast in my clinic
was a highlight all-right

Chapter
twelve

THE FINAL FIGHT I had with my wife was when four years ago I drove with my brother Rob to Sydney to support an exhibition of recent paintings by Bill Hay, a friend since 1976 when I bumped into him pumping his bike up hard outside St Kilda West Post Office, and we've been close friends since that chance meeting, or pumping. I didn't tell my wife Rob was going to Sydney with me because they've never got on. I filled the car with unleaded and bought cigarettes and mineral water and straight into the desert we went.

The weather temperate, the conversation comical, we marvelled at the same boring hills we marvelled at thirty-eight years earlier. The sunlight and the dying stockman, et cetera. We propped at a tenth-rate motel for $100 a night including insomnia and he snored so loudly I sat up stupid all night wishing I were alone. His adenoids were not the best. That and his chainsmoking.

That night we both showered, and dined in the restaurant of that infernal motel near Goulburn. There was something seriously defunct about the air-conditioning and the dining room smelled of fan-forced excrement in vast amounts, most noticeably when the food was served up. The dining room was decorated with sorrow. The guests seemed sarcophagi. Rubber bread rolls, frozen butter pats and rigor mortis. Appalling nylon Afghani carpets and vinyl otter on the wall. We chose the Brown Brothers white to start and their idea of red to end. Luckily you could smoke in there so we both did and really enjoyed that as it was free. We ate fatty local beef, six millimetres in width, and gnawed indifferently upon the spring onion.

That night we drank more in the room and talked, watching the cheap dark. In the morning I had a go at him for his insistent adenoidal snoring but he quite justifiably accused me of loud snoring too; in fact he said it was louder than his cacophonies of interrupted breathing.

We motored on past Goulburn, wearying of the sepia landscape of more hills than you could poke a twig at until the car expired at Gunning. I was going down a great hill at 125 kph when all the panel lights came on in a very alarming way. The engine stalled and I had to pull over without steering because the steering stalled when the engine did. Quite a manufacturing hiccup, that.

To our luck we made it into a ditch by the edge of a clearing or an abyss of some sort. Old cobwebbed semi-trailer recaps strewn off trucks lay forsaken down the bottom of it in rubberised ruin. 'I wonder why the Corolla stopped like that?' he said, sitting with me on the road.

'I've no idea,' I answered. 'None, whatever!'

After letting the hot engine have a cool-down for half an hour I lifted up the bonnet for a look-see. What on earth would I know or care about cars? The radiator was fizzing with unparalleled heat and the battery had foamed at its mouth since we left dear Goulburn.

No way would it start and I very nearly bent the thin ignition key by violent repeated turnings in the stupid and stubborn ignition-barrel. It got hot, very. The sun blazed down upon the two moron brothers. The engine of the car looked quite put out, which was distressing. The tyres were all sort of scorched and so on.

Did this story contribute to the hole in my marriage? I think it did, now that I think about my stupidity, my errant stupidity: my wife used to say when we fought, 'You *deliberately* and *wilfully* misunderstand things.' I am wilful and obstinate and life goes contrary with me. It depresses me that I am intelligent but unintelligent.

My brother chainsmoked in this horrid gulch and his bottom sat on a hot truck tyre that had split on the Hume Highway due to expansion in the heat and now was home to toads and the like. Robbo was all red in the face and just smoked one after the other. I flagged down a pair of gay cyclists as they came together down the hill where my vehicle had just expired. They wore the same kinds of expensive sunglasses and trendy vinyl hallucinatory yellow T-shirts. They reluctantly stopped.

After yabbering away in the ferocious heat they telephoned help. They rang on their mobiles and the New South Wales interpretation of Victoria's RACV got there in an hour, or was supposed to get there, but they didn't. We thanked the generous cyclists who parked their shiny bums in the air and sped off. Rob used his last minute's worth of credit to ring the RACV in Melbourne and after sixty-nine seconds' worth of muzak he was put through to a voice-chip that assured him my car wasn't covered. I couldn't afford Roadside Assistance and as a result I'd lapsed. Consequently no assistance could be expected from their interstate colleagues. It was forty degrees and we had no water nor food to absorb; only the guaranteed information that we were in deep shit. We stayed there all day.

Towards five in the afternoon an impressive running-on-twenty-cylinders compactor came along, which had Beethoven playing in double dolby in its cabin; the drivers liked him. It had air-conditioning and a bar, you name it. The guy rang a tow-truck operator based at Tahmoor, 100 kilometres from Sydney, near Picton. It was a hair-raising ride in the cabin of the silent but efficient tow-truck man. He disobeyed the speed-limits and ran lights and never explained just where we both were or where Tahmoor happened to be. I was starving and so was poor Rob.

In the end we arrived at fly-infested country Tahmoor and the tow-truck man charged us two hundred bucks for his effort; I had three hundred in cash in my jeans-pocket, so forked nearly all of it over. He wheeled off in a pong of hot rubber with just a whiff of laughter, I thought.

The old motor-mechanic guy smoked as he undid the hot bonnet for a look. I was pretty alarmed the way he smoked right on top of the carburettor and prayed that nothing bad would happen or my car go up in exciting flames, but nothing happened.

After a whole lot of inspection and guesswork he said it was fucked. We had to leave it at Tahmoor and hope he was honest, and he was, as it transpired, at least he fixed it in the end, but it took him four days to nut out exactly what happened to the normally reliable car. Rob and I caught the train into Central Railway Station and headed to Surry Hills where Ray Hughes showed Bill's paintings. They weren't there.

That particular walk we did from Central to Ray Hughes Gallery in Devonshire Street, Surry Hills, was arduous for a few reasons. First off it was unbearably humid, hotter than any previous body heat experienced by me, and I have been to Malacca, where at fifty-four degrees my thongs melted. Although vastly muggy and fearfully evaporative the night's weather also included monstrous hailstones mixed with sheet lightning and barrels of thunder. It commenced to rain as well as stay furnace-like, and anyway we made it to the gallery and went on to an Indian restaurant where Ray had said they'd be if they'd gone from his gallery. No one in it.

We wandered the tiresome drag of boring Surry Hills for hours trying to find them, but no Indian café included any of them for their opening night bash. In the end we legged it to Kings Cross, carting bags of clothing and hanging out for a drink. I bought a bottle of cold champagne made in Edenhope, and we drank it in the gutter and felt much revived.

I rented a small crypt for ninety a night and forked over the full rent so at least we both had a roof over our heads. I didn't want to sleep out in seedy Kings Cross. Cats raped dogs there. We had a shower and bought botulism burgers. We ate them and drank beer till we fell into a deep repose and snored in tandem. It was perfectly right what my young brother had claimed about me snoring as bad as him, for I woke at three in the morning due to my new apnea and heard myself snore, and loud it was. I apologised to my brother in my sleep. God, I slept great after that grog and all that walking around saturated Sydney. I ached all over but slept like a kid.

In the morning we breakfasted on cheap runny eggs and cardiac-arrest bacon for four dollars each man, including imitation mango juice that was secretly made of oranges. We had lots of black coffee and hit Hyde Park and really enjoyed the mystical sight of the old Moreton Bay fig trees in whose trunks I've observed carvings of comical ogres and ghastly gnarled grey witches beckoning to me. We went over to Ray Hughes Gallery and not one painting had sold. Bill is a fantastic painter but that's how it goes at times; I've known it too from my shows that haven't sold a single caricature.

We tucked into a yum cha and a few laughs and Rob and I went back to the backpackers' slum where our soggy stuff was. It was still so muggy that all this black came out in me. Like soot or treacle or pollution or just bad karma. The trip to Sydney was an unmitigated disaster. I felt like Napoleon invading Russia.

I rang my wife on Rob's mobile, which he'd put a few bucks on, but she couldn't have cared less about my travails. She was cold as ice. She said I ought to have paid my RACV Roadside levies and been current before choofing off to Sydney like that. She said I never planned ahead and brought the entire catastrophe on myself. I was aghast.

There was either porn or loneliness in the Cross, take your pick. We looked at a Rembrandt retrospective but, as Rob pointed out, he's dead. We drank in bars and smoked and walked around like two golliwogs in mugginess. We saw a play at the Nimrod Theatre, which was appalling. *Anne Frank on Ice.* It was an ice-capade in bad taste.

After our so-called holiday we caught the train to antique Tahmoor again as we missed it so. The guy was as he was when first he appeared as a line drawing of a bush mechanic in bib and brace overalls covered in axle grease and a hangover, leaning his lined visage over the carburettor with a whole lot of ash cascading off his smoke, looking intently into the various tubing and coiled unfathomable detail of a car that won't start.

We had to endure the entire day in inbred Tahmoor, where all the townsfolk looked like cartoons of incestuous bush types. Uglier than mud on a fence, they were up that way. We went into the pub and thousands of big fat flies accompanied Rob as he went in to use the toilet, if a chap were caught doing wee in a lane in Tahmoor they'd hang you. It was a reactionary place, Tahmoor. I was told by the redneck barkeep it cost a buck to use the lavatory and all his henchmen started giggling in a high falsetto way. I bought a packet of matches in order to pay symbolically for my brother urinating as he had been hanging on all day, he whined, and was desperate for a drop in bowel-pressure that can really be terribly uncomfortable.

Ten hours of hanging round Tahmoor. Nothing on the television in the pub but the Melbourne Cup. We backed a loser each way and wandered back to the garage to see if after six days the guy could get me going again. He showed me Japanese artwork of the 1990 Corolla and a heap of computerised information to do with my car's electronic wizardry. I couldn't follow anything no matter how he raved. I wrote him out a cheque for $690 and drove back to Melbourne immediately, with Rob looking hung over and all red-eyed and generally we didn't look the best.

There were these magnificent real boulders that went up to the sky, vast chasms and endless nuclear bridges and power plants and future technology gone mad and cacti.

Fifty kilometres out of Tahmoor on the Hume Highway the right wiper came off during an impromptu rainstorm; the rubber squeegee that's connected to its waving aluminium arm came away completely and the metal rod of the right wiper got snagged in the windscreen rubber on the outside of the car, so I couldn't see a thing, then it hailstormed hard as possible.

We easily could have, or ought to have, been killed during the ensuing weather chaos. There was no way I could really peer properly through the unsqueegeed right-hand side of the front car windscreen as the idiotic right wiper-arm had by now completely slid out of its metal housing and lay draped across the screen snagged upon my rearview mirror. It was alarming to say the least.

Rob read the paper, checked his zodiac and in a rather relaxed fashion completed the *Daily Telegraph*'s crossword puzzle. 'What is a four-letter word for trouble?' he screamed through the quite loud claps of thunder.

My wife was exasperated with over two and three-quarter decades of recklessness and un-insightfulness that always landed us in that four-letter word for stress Rob was reading about.

I am too fickle and too wilful and over-excited by the sheer romance of finding myself animate. I have tried to temper these fatal flaws with my writing.

But the gulf between writing and reality is fatal if you don't watch out. It is all very well to respond to adventures and sally forth if one is unmarried and without children, but one of my major faults is the spontaneous abandonment of meditation upon possible outcomes, and the rapid approval of harebrained action. Just like Toad in *Wind in the Willows*.

I am quite certain it was the Tahmoor Disaster that contributed to my downfall. It was a bit rash, the whole miserable saga of wrongful brain energy married with the determination of pleasure. The joy was selfish and dangerous but seemed at the time a surrealistic film.

For some reason known only to the fates it began to get hot after eight in the evening, most hot, in fact awful. I filled the tank in Albury and rang my wife, who was out with our son, having written me off. I rang her mobile and only received her recorded message saying she wasn't available at the moment.

Near Seymour I got stuck between a convoy of trucks we once called semi-trailers and they kept my car wedged between them tight. It was teeming down raining and the windscreen kept badly fogging up and the demister didn't work so I kept reaching out and vigorously rubbing the inside of the windscreen with my own unsteering hand in order to see nothing but red tail-lights all in a row.

I tried a couple of times to get around this stifling mass of trucks and put the right indicator on and felt the momentary thrill of going somewhere, instead of remaining stuck in limbo, but that truck only slowed and braked to curtail the overtaking plan. In short it was dangerous.

I pulled over at a ghost town where it was said Ned Kelly was born; it's called Beveridge and was almost to Melbourne so we bought a burger and rested. The trucks were braying and endless and the city was nuclear and vast; so vast and completely different from the small place, or so it seemed to me, when I was a boy growing up in its charms and borrowed accents and little dusty bookshops.

As I sipped the gluggy, tasteless, imitation rat-dropping coffee from the timeless polystyrene foam takeaway beaker and sat with my brother Rob on the side of the road, which at least took us out of traffic and confusing noises such as the demented mooing of doomed cows en route to an interesting slaughterhouse and sudden arrivals of fiery bits of discarded truck tyre cast off the trucks due to their fatigue, which could decapitate a motorist or hitchhiker, I remembered my teenage years.

Sipping the joke coffee it came to me that before I signed up to write about my strange place of birth and agreed to describe it in play or poem on page, my life when it was young was carefree and happy. My parents were happy and worked eagerly at their stuff, he doing the printing, she the housework, my three happy brothers and I were a squad of joy.

I loved working hard like my father did; I got up at a quarter to five in the morning and rode my bike over to Mr Haldayne, the Reservoir newspaper shop proprietor, and all the kids stuffed their sugar bags with fresh newspapers and delivered them to people irrespective of whether they felt like bad news or not. People adore bad news. Mr Haldayne worshipped bad news. It paid his home off. He was a short, tenacious, wiry sort of man who wore a crisply dry-cleaned dustcoat and bicycle leggings to keep his trouser cuffs out of the greasy chain as he pedalled nonchalantly to Eternity. He was born pedalling.

The shop he had was a farce. It was littered with sleepy boys with twelve years' worth of life who were either gifted at folding in half fresh copies of the *Sun News-Pictorial* or *The Age*, which fitted on either side of your sewn-up sugarbag with a split in it to sit over what was called a 'horse', which was a strange-looking saddle affair that went over the main bar of your bike. It was wobbly, in a way, to start pedalling with that thing on you.

Mr Haldayne had grey, stiff, beaver-like fur for his hair and in fact he looked beaver all over. He talked to himself loudly all the time, always adding the words, 'He said' to each originating phlegmatic sentence, so he sounded like, 'How are you today, young Dickins, he said. Oh, darn it, there I go again adding, "He said" again, he said.' He was nuts.

I thought then by the side of the road which led to what was once called my place, of all the places I've stayed, written in, all the girlfriends and desks and bad prose and decent prose, all the faux pas and sessions on the wine bottle, often as not for no other reason than to wind down and fall asleep to fell the tinkering restless brain, but the occasional drink is no excuse for slovenliness of one's spirit.

Fancy risking both our lives going up to Sydney like that on a whim only to break down in Tahmoor, New South Wales, and put the marriage over the line. It was never the same after Tahmoor, a real landmark in my ruin. She said, 'You never grow up.'

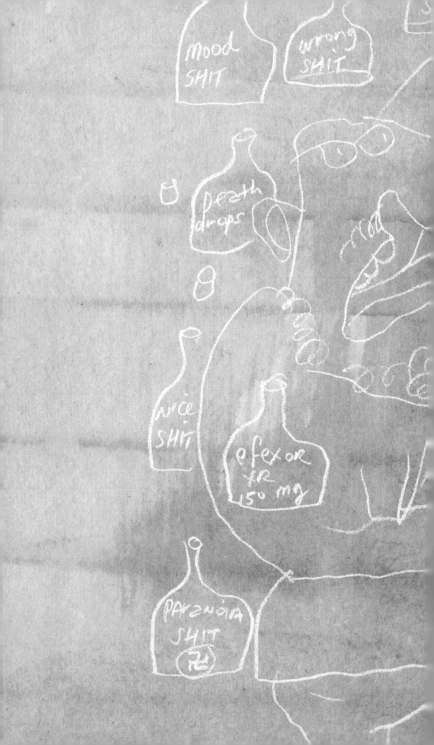

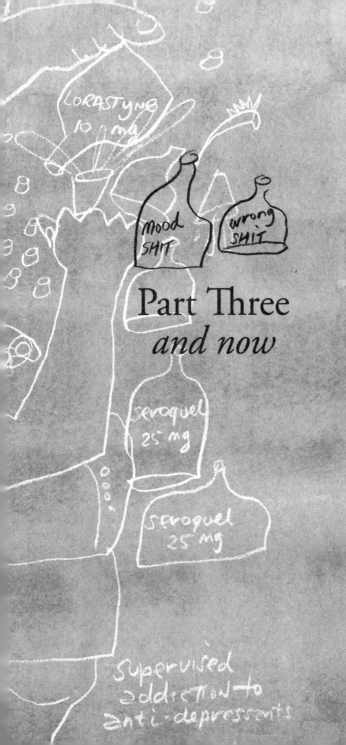

Part Three
and now

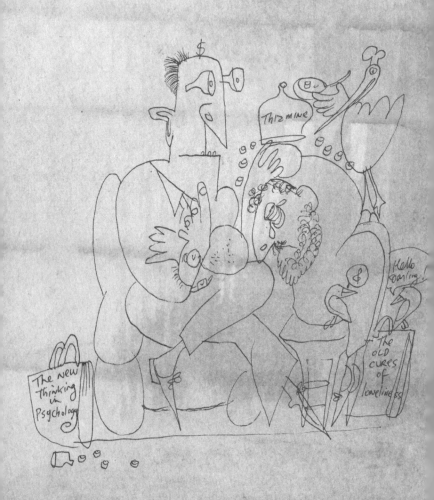

Chapter
one

THE QUIRKY THING about depression is that when you are finally cleared of the clinic you wander in a drugged manner into the city where every single person you encounter is completely and utterly insane. It's a big clinic. It is springtime in Melbourne now and you'd expect folks to be friendlier merely because the weather is so luscious. They are not. It's a world of egomaniacs who loathe everybody else as soon as they detect them or hear them or smell them so suspiciously.

I lived in a motel for a fortnight after I got out of the clinic; for lots of those nights my boy Lou slept right by in his single bed and I in my one near the window. He made sure I took my medication every single evening after we ate out. I tried to cook for us both one night but failed because the tiny motel room only had a Cambodian microwave in it with Cambodian settings I couldn't quite follow.

To Louis's stupefaction his father tried to heat chilli baked beans like we saw on the telly but they just got real gluggy and sort of warm on the exterior only stone-cold in the centre of them. Even when Daddy added sauce they were frightful. He scraped his into the bin but I devoured mine. We were both of us dreadfully disciplined at the horrid motel in Arden Street.

I think the oddest thing that happened there in that cramped dump that management charged $88 a night to be safe in was the morning John Cain rang me, the former Victorian Labor premier. 'It's John Cain here, Barry.' He wanted me to read some poetry a junkie had composed while relaxing at Her Majesty's Jail out at Barwon. I wonder how he got my motel number? I didn't give it to him.

A few weeks after we bade forlorn goodbyes to that motel, I discovered a cottage in North Carlton and signed a year's lease.

My art-teacher friend Heather Lee read the article Graham Reilly ran in *The Age* about my experience with depression, then she made up a multicoloured box containing bottles of food dye and pencils and sable-hair watercolour brushes. She posted it to me and when I was out I opened it and she had added an envelope.

When I nervously undid it I saw she had written: 'My dear friend of many decades, as a fellow art teacher when I read your article in the "Opinion" section of *The Age* today I felt benumbed! That you of all people, who have amused Melburnians with articles and books and plays and been on television and the radio for years – that you of all people should suffer like that…!'

She added, 'And Barry, you *will* paint!' I ventured out into the micro-lonely paved courtyard and made a start at once.

Food dye is fantastic to work with; the colours are literally out of this world, I have to say, particularly the purple and the vermilion red, not to mention the incandescent yellow that appears bright orange in its humble jar but when you splash some cold water onto it, it goes crazy. Brighter than Van Gogh's yellows, and weren't they something?

Having got myself weaned off the drugs set for me at the clinic I now don't sleep very well, lucky to get a few hours but so what? I'm sixty soon. At least I'm not medicated anymore. And the tiny bit of natural repose feels better than drugged unconsciousness does. I say that as a sage veteran of both.

I arise in the wee hours of the late November morning and put on the electric kettle. I gave a hundred for that trendy kettle at a beastly electric goods shop in dreary Clifton Hill. The guy who sold it to me was a word I don't use.

I sip Nescafé instant cappuccino in the frigid courtyard and let loose with the hyperenergetic food dye at two in the morning. I buy the very best watercolour paper I can afford and when the accidental colours are lying in vivid pools doing their stuff, I wait for the effect to dry bone-hard and go inside to write, either this or that manuscript or an article for the newspaper.

When the big sheet of watercolour paper is unquestionably bone-dry, which can take all day if the weather is bad, I go back into it with an array of charcoal pencils, willow charcoal that breaks too easily, but then again that is possibly due to the fact I am so passionate about drawing. I use white chalk and grey chalk and Chinograph pencils that are of wax and are meant to use on celluloid but are nifty for the details I want. One picture last week took sixty hours to set right. I sold it for $500 and got the rent.

I never bother anymore with the concept of sleep or fretting. I just got myself nice and relaxed doing something I have always adored. Drawing. I am fifty-nine but the same happy boy my dad showed how to draw half a century ago. I never show *my* boy one of my pictures these days, as that would be an unnecessary pressure on him. Fathers shouldn't look for praise anywhere but in the fridge where the mayonnaise is kept. I am working towards a new exhibition.

Each morning I walk up Lee Street to buy the newspaper. Often as not I quite wonder why I bother to read it when you can just as easily read children's faces and realise life has meaning, whereas mass-circulation meanness has no life. I return home with it under my arm and drink Nescafé and read about death or pole-vaulting. I then wish I had a table in my courtyard to paint pictures with.

Unluckily, for art one requires a table to begin watercolour painting with, otherwise your powders and saucepans full of water tend to get knocked over by your clumsy feet. For two months I awoke and instantly painted without a table, there being none. I knelt like a praying mantis and used the charcoal on the kitchen floor. It's a bugger when a breadcrumb gets under the paper and you muck the picture up. I suppose you call painting on the floor, if it's a large work, a floral or even a floor-al. As opposed to a mural. I drift.

Those heavenly early strolls to the disillusioning Seven-Eleven were paramount for my collective consciousness, even if I were unconscious. The not-bad French Romantic landscape painter Corot used to say he felt fantastic up early. There is something gorgeous about bus fumes and cyclists blaspheming.

Coming home from that gloomy shop, one day I paused to patiently contemplate this beautiful old 1920s Baltic pine table in Lee Street, Carlton, that just about talked to me in its anthropomorphic uniqueness. It smiled, if old wood can, and said it adored me madly.

I felt the same way for it, of course, and ran my eyes over its creamy surface. It even had a 1920 penny attached to its passive front, not glued for that would be pornographic, but inlaid artistically somehow by some long-ago loving artisan's hand, to show the year of its creation. It had crude cobalt blue octopus straps wrapped around its legs and was tightly tethered to a big black cast-iron fence 130 years old.

Everything about it was bliss, potential and wonder. It was a desk for all seasons, but especially late November in north Carlton, where my spirit blossomed. I used to wonder if that table would ever be mine, but surely that's too hopeful in an age of distrust, despair and cruelty. It proved too taxing to paint my watercolours on the slippery kitchen floor; my back used to give out.

A week ago the guy whose table it was came out of his terrace and said to me, 'If you stare at my table anymore you'll wear it out.' I felt suitably rebuked and made to walk off, but then he added as a postscript, 'Would you like it?' As the hippies used to say, that blew my mind. Who gives away anything but morbidity these days? He does. He and his friend carried it round to my battered back gate. They lifted it over the jammed stubborn gate, which can't open unless you give it a hearty kick. They set it down and I didn't know how to thank them. They didn't require thanks. They were kind.

I went to see Jim, my old publican mate who owns the Lomond Hotel in Nicholson Street, and asked him what was the finest claret available. He suggested a drop from McLaren Vale in South Australia. He said it was as nice as you can get anywhere at all. I bought it at once and gave it to the friendly neighbours who gave me the free table. By chance they had friends over for dinner, they said, and we shook hands in their doorway.

They have moved now and the table has moved too, into my daily dreams of mixing up food dyes and acids and reactive substances such as hope and ecstasy. Now the perplexity of depression waxes and wanes like the unpredictability of dreams or psalms that I paint at dawn when the birds sing just for me. When the brightest colours I can make start to dry out like alcoholics in the morning light. When the first bells can be detected from Lee Street Primary School. And the happy little innocent children run into class like tumbling love poems.

I didn't expect kindness from a couple of strangers like that.

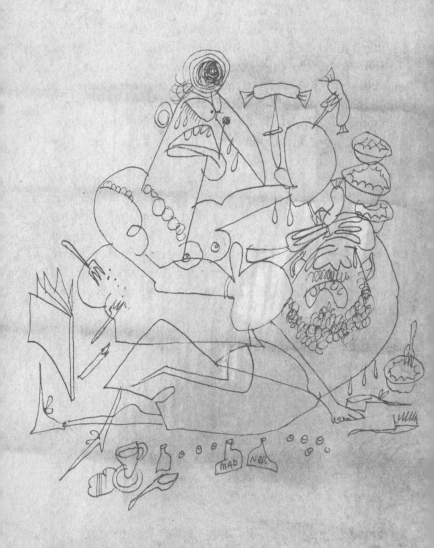

Chapter
two

NOT LONG BACK I played tennis with my son Lou in the Fitzroy courts of time gone by. The breeze was so refreshing I foolishly felt I'd live forever. My son adores tennis; I am getting on and he's heading for fourteen. We're friends. He doesn't judge me. But he is put out when I offer him a begrimed dinner plate if I run out of Korean tea towels. He studies the plates like an Egyptian lapis-lazuli jeweller: 'Ah, grime!'

Lou served well, putting a lot of top spin on some of the first serves so they curled memorably; he likes coming in to the net and volleying, so he beat me a lot.

The ancient trees in the gardens seemed alive again as if they too just got over clinical depression, and they positively bloomed in their jades and emeralds, and possums scampered up their fossilised bark and I smelt flowers again and got my first serve in and remembered the psychiatrist assuring me I was deteriorating. 'There is no doubt you are deteriorating,' he used to say at our useless interviews. No wonder I was deteriorating, as well as demoralised and demonised.

As we ran around on the courts and lobbed and chipped away and top-spinned and drop-shotted and the sun came out, the sweaty guy next door, I mean the court to my left, was swearing and grunting and putting me off using intemperate language. Try as I might I couldn't block him out and his blaspheming only got worse and his swearing got louder and he proved so distracting to me I just couldn't concentrate. He and his partner just belted the ball with such masculinity I couldn't see my own tennis ball properly. Then a very loud Italian tennis coach a few courts away put me off too. I started to become anxious as though it was just masculinity that was the problem.

A week into the beginning of my new rental life in my small hut my son was watching television; I was in the courtyard working on a big new chalk and food-dye drawing for a new show. The phone in the bedroom rang shrilly, so my son answered it. It was my wife. He put me on and instantly we quarrelled, heatedly over some trifling matter, not trifling to her on the other end, but it was an arrangement where she wanted me to do something I really didn't feel like. Because we hadn't been getting on, the voices went up in volume and I found myself speaking in some sort of weird way, funny that. We started to shout on the telephone – I can't remember why – and the son got on the phone after a couple of minutes' worth of abuse, and he wanted me to get out of the bedroom and I think he pushed at the door in a groping, sort of blind, frightened way due to the sheer emotionalism of the fight between his mum and dad, then for some reason he sat at my writing-desk and started frantically to write his feelings out in pen on paper.

He wept furiously; his sweet angelic face cried like a fountain and his writing hand tore at his literature. He wrote so hard his forming words bit straight through the crumpled A4 paper. Then he was using a new fine-liner I had bought at Officeworks but his burning-hot cascading tears of frustration blurred all his words anyway. His new essay on loneliness just ran away onto the cheap carpet and his runners. I was right in his way, right in the way of his young straight body writing furiously down the emotions he was sensing and as he scribbled the words on the saturated A4 pages he barked at me to 'get out the room!' He wanted to be alone and sort out the matter with his mother on the phone. I hate phones.

Then two days later she telephoned me or I telephoned her and to my stupefaction she wept when we spoke, and she said she couldn't stop worrying about me, that she thought I 'might go back in' again, meaning the clinic but that would never occur again in my life.

I would kill myself first. I told her I knew I couldn't be lived with. She spoke in a gentle, concerned way and in the end I started cracking a few jokes and telling a few light-hearted accounts of things I'd seen in the street, prelude to my drawings that were really abstractions and dreams of reality seen through chalk and watercolours. The latest pictures are quite large; as are my latest tears. I'm learning to cry in 3D.

Then one day in the rental property, I was talking to her about something trivial and insignificant, just raving away but she seemed sort of connected, then I looked into her eyes, which I know like the lines I have written for my plays and I realised she was weeping, possibly with boredom but more likely sadness that we were over. I said, 'There must be some part of you that still loves me.' She answered, 'Of course there is.' I tried to hold her but it didn't comfort her much and like the great satirist she is, she muttered like Groucho Marx, 'This is just so uncomfortable for me.' And we both briefly laughed.

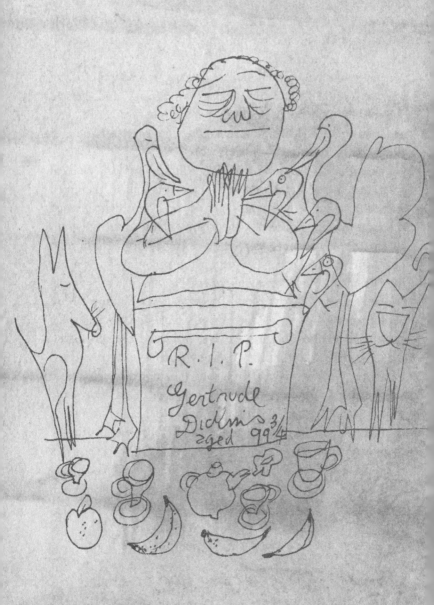

R.I.P.
Gertrude
Dickins
aged 99¾

Chapter
three

SOMEONE STOLE my cheap mobile telephone recently after my son and I came home from Chinatown, where we dined together, he upon Peking chicken and me on sharkfin soup. The mobile is worth thirty-nine bucks at Crazy Johns. I have been using it for a few months but don't understand it. Wilful. I can't see the little numbers to hit any of them to get through to anyone I know. My fingertips mis-hit the invisible digits so I telephone people I don't know, which I think is against the law; in fact I'm sure it is.

I backtracked our steps and revisited the tennis courts, where it seemed to lie near the darkening umpire's stand. The courts were padlocked. You could scale the fence but there was menacing barbed wire atop. I didn't need to either castrate myself or just hang there. I then remembered I had the mobile with me at the Chinatown café. I had a short-term memory loss of it lying next to my sharkfin soup.

So I choofed into Chinatown and parked half a mile from the same café as I didn't want to get booked. The proprietor looked in a bored way through his drawer but said no one had handed it in. Was it all the ECT shots that made me lose my memory? Was it or wasn't it? No matter where in my new rented half-house I searched there was no trace. I even looked on top of the little toilet in the courtyard, which is where I leave it. I leave it there out of punishment as it 'dings' too much for my liking.

I rang my brother Rob to ring my mobile in order to hear it go off, but that ingenious idea didn't work. I spent all of Tuesday ringing employers and friends giving them my mobile number but then I realised someone had pinched it. It had three cents worth of credit left so the robber wouldn't have been able to ring many people; certainly not overseas.

I drove to Crazy Johns in Sydney Road and two highly conscientious girls spent ninety minutes putting my existing mobile number on a new Chinese mobile telephone and cancelled the old pinched mobile telephone. They were kind to me, extremely. I was grateful to them both and decided to give them twenty bucks apiece as a reward for their patience.

Ever since the electroconvulsive treatments my short-term memory is not dependable and it is so upsetting. I walk around with my car and house keys in my hand for fear they will walk. I am forever losing my savings book from my bank. They won't give you a new one if you lose the old one. I've been lectured before about that.

I'd always been absentminded but never like this. My wife astonished me a month back when in the car she said very quietly it was nine times I'd had ECT. I thought it was six. I was staggered it was that much. My wife and I have been not getting on for a year; you need to have been apart for a year to actually divorce.

Nowadays she sleeps in the silt of her renovating terrace house, dines on dust the renovators create, chokes upon the plaster filings that dwindle down, in her way she intends the loafing builders to feel guilty she is there while they do it everlastingly.

One afternoon I went back to our old home, the trace of

130 years in leafy Carlton, and she was teaching and so not there; our cat was, so I patted it, then up the dusty stairs I went and very nearly plummeted through a pair of missing steps the builder had reason to remove but not replace, just a yawning chasm of about thirty feet to the lounge room floor. Not a bad way to die, I suppose.

My poor, honest, hard-working wife asleep in plaster dust a third of an inch thick while the builder works on another home he has not told us about; that is why he is so snail-like. She has to live for many months in filth and ashes and her hip is killing her and I keep on going to the chemist shop to buy her painkillers that do not work, not even a whole packet.

Home was never the million-buck terrace we lived in for ten years in Carlton. It is a place where you don't fight. It is peace and school sandwiches and a nightly match of tennis between my son and me in the twilight Fitzroy tennis courts, where I played when I was really young like him. Home is a meal not spilt or milk not choked on and sleep without alcohol in it or cigarettes in it or unrest in it or bad moods in it. Just toast and marg and contented snoring.

Recently, at eight in the morning of a calm Sunday, my wife telephoned to inform me she wanted to take our son to church; really she just wanted to be with him on a Sunday. He stayed at my place and when he awoke I presented him with a fresh punnet of strawberries for his breakfast, which I left on his armchair as he watched the 'toons. I am trying not to pressure him to eat more fruit than crisps, which he's hooked on, like all kids. It was a small, informal, lazy Sunday morning world of longed-for-laziness and we both didn't want to go anywhere, do anything or say a single syllable to each other. 'I just want lazy time, Mummy,' he said.

I sipped a coffee in the breezy courtyard and had a hay-fevered look at the paper, realising once again nothing is funny. It was just fantastic not to rush around like a hairy goat for once, as that is the mainstay of my day. Rushing to chat to schools to obtain part-time poetry-teaching, rushing to be stood up at a fashionable café, rushing to park and shop just like all of us on earth. She came in and they were gone in an instant. I started writing for a few hours but then felt empty because I hadn't anticipated her arrangements, which are always spontaneous. Is this our future as separated parents of a thirteen-year-old boy? To quarrel over arrangements?

I have to be a new man. Bright and magnanimous, and things will go well. I don't want to sign up with the constantly growing army of tough guys, never forgiving while such forces like forgiveness are powerful and can make you kind. I recall her coming into the clinic so frequently, after nine hours in the school and all the heavy traffic and the pick-ups. What must I have been like to live with? Exhausting, probably; definitely full of myself, welded to the egomaniacal passion to upstage and earbash. My whingeing became an art form. She must have felt used-up and a bit bitterer.

Now I am weaned off anti-depressants and going ahead with what my GP instructed me to do after my release. 'Take eight weeks as though you're still in the clinic and take the lot at night at whatever home you're in and after two months go off them.' I have done this and feel like the old self again before all the selves divvied up to destroy me.

My melancholy lifts; this afternoon I met Pamela Bakes, who runs an antique bookshop in Fitzroy and it was like meeting a woman of my vintage and background but she was just so easy to talk to and she says she'll type up a play I am writing on Dylan Thomas for Richard Piper, who is a splendid actor. She said she believes in random acts of kindness. This is one of them. I'm going to give her one of my latest big chalk and colour drawings. Just seeing her made me believe in people again.

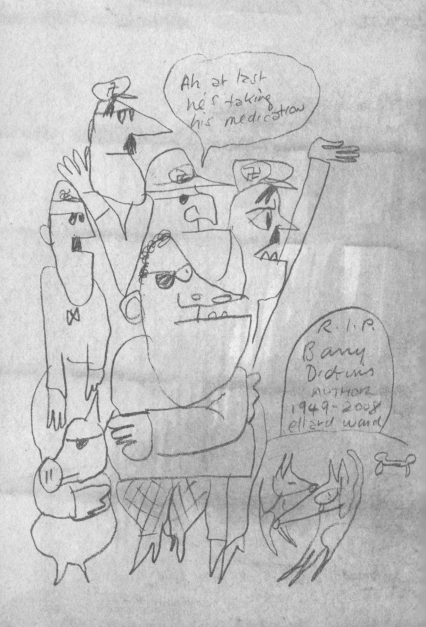

Chapter
four

Last Saturday Lou and I got up at six to prepare for the evils of Saint Michael's Under Fourteen Tennis Club in Lalor, about an hour out of Melbourne if you make it through a sea of abattoir trucks. Louis sipped a large orange juice squeezed in Christmas Island by refugees. He watched the 'toons and leapt into the Corolla. We picked up his gangly team-mates at Fitzroy Tennis Club in the accumulated November weathers of our city, very muggy and ice-cold, a hundred degrees and subsequently below zero. I put my enlargers on my great big nose to study the street directory as you'd study Mozart's *Requiem*. It was incredibly difficult to find Saint Michael's in Lalor. You had to be a genius.

I executed a big felt pen drawing of how to get there but the breeze puffed it out the window, the tennis children silent at that ghastly hour in my bomb car with two bucks' worth of gas in it, I knew to follow Plenty Road.

I bought one sullen boy a chocolate jam donut and he ate it without commentary in the back; I could overhear his thankless jaw working on its interior helium. We pulled up and went in to be ignored by Saint Michael's. No hi and no goodbye when they won, and we left in silence.

It is the new order of things never to be greeted or said hello to after an hour's ride through suburban hell. No one asked, 'Did you find us okay?' or 'Didn't get lost, did you, in Plenty Road on the way out here?' No one spoke and when I asked in a polite way if I could have a coffee to wake up a bit, this woman said in a shrill way, 'Just a second, would you!' She was engaged in the ancient art of sponging rain out of saturated artificial lawn tennis courts with a funny-looking sponge-roller you drag along while looking displeased. Some pimply Saint Michael's kids were playing ping-pong in the ugly clubhouse with bats with only half the plywood handle on them and a dint in the ping-pong ball. My son was keen to play too but they hogged it.

It was eight in the morning in late November 2008 and my starving son and shivery me gnawed on a frozen KitKat in the parked Corolla. The lady who ran the outfit took forty minutes to organise the first set even though the courts were dry enough to hit the ball on. At the rear of Saint Michael's were more courts made out of en-tout-cas, which I'd never learnt to pronounce or spell. Our kids weren't invited to have a warm-up. Our kids weren't allowed to have anything, and had to hang around; it was three degrees and supposed to be summer. I had a chip of the ball with Louis in the car park and it felt good just to move your legs a bit in such melancholic weather conditions. You expected seals to slither by.

Because a father in our team called Willem seeds the five kids in the squad, my son only played one game of singles, and waited with his icicled companions by the Auschwitz tennis-court fence to try to look through it to see who was winning. In the Saint Michael's clubhouse there were lots of caterers' cans of Nescafé but no one offered the other parents and me a single spoonful of it to try to wake up with at that early hour. Their faces were as if dead.

I saw one tall, freak, youngish Saint Michael's player rolling the sponge-thing over the artificial grass to squeegee the moisture out of it that had bucketed down overnight; he was over six foot in height and I was later told only thirteen years of age, all puss-pimples yet to erupt on his sourpuss face that could only have been conceived in godforsaken Lalor. He looked like he didn't give a hoot, which naturally enough, he did not, about anything. Not refugees, not anything. He wilfully squeegeed the court with a royal sneer. He wore expensive sunglasses and reminded me of the prison officer in *Cool Hand Luke*, who is in awe of the Paul Newman character's rebelliousness and panache but acts completely indifferent anyway, in true Lalor style. I called out to him from the sort-of-porch where we sat to watch the children play: 'Do you know what time the kids get started, please, mate?' He said something incomprehensible and kept sullenly squeegeeing.

I was so desperately sleepy and didn't want to be that way to watch my son play his singles, so I rebelliously slid undone the giant family Lalor tin of Nescafé and shoved a tablespoon of it into a cup and in bliss sipped the revolting muck you need to wake up with, otherwise you turn into Harpo. The great, big, young, pimply kid who had just rolled the artificial grass court was now 'versing' against some other team of little kids from the northern suburbs, and had a strange circus hammer action in respect of his first serve. He just chucked the ball up and hit the shit out of it. It was the hardest I have ever seen anything struck in my life. In my brief and long fifty-nine years I have witnessed many things hit pretty hard, including myself, but that lout hit that clout harder. Much, much harder, it was a revelatory blow. Smoke, though invisible, came off the ball.

My son observed this hard-smitten tennis ball and whirled his eager and gentle angelic face to me and whispered confidentially to me in an undertone so no Saint Michael personage could possibly hear him, 'Gee, Daddles, did you see how hard that guy in the sunglasses just hit the first serve?' We almost laughed but held our composure. You're not to laugh at anything there. Full stop.

I felt old and thirteen at Saint Michael's last Saturday morning in the three degrees of separation. You only need another three degrees to go insane. The aggro parents, be they Afghani or Anglo-Saxon. Lalor lived only for its children winning. No courtesies, no niceties and no shaking hands at the net and saying, 'Bad luck or good luck or anything except we hate you.' The cold sleepy parents coached their depressed but assertive children out there in mosquito-bearing conditions; it was a hundred thousand weathers all screwed up in Lalor, the thermals altered all the time, mozzies were born in the netting; they kept the net in the fridge at Saint Michael's.

My son was the only player who was calm. He looked like the chosen one in the middle of the marvellous Bosch of a sublimely peaceful angel in an ocean of ogres. My son is just so happy to be around. The mere fact of his finding himself alive each day turns him on. I am just like him, a thing in me that annoys people who demand conventional behaviour. His unsurprised joy in finding himself being not just alive but also a spokesperson for life is beyond any measure. He is the spirit of unqualified joy as much as he is the unqualified symbol of happiness.

Beacon to me in the unsure dark, he waits for me on the sun-flayed nature strip outside his high school and the happiness seeps into my car. I've had the 1990 white Corolla ten years, my only possession apart from my 1989 fibreglass dentures paid off in 1990, made by hand in Collins Street by Doctor Star.

When Louis turned ten a few years back his mother baked him his favourite citric wholemeal spongecake and we celebrated at La Porcella Restaurant in Rathdowne Street. We dined on scrumptious roast quail and laughed a lot and my wife and I sang him 'Happy Birthday' at about ten at night. We lit sparklers on his cake and he sipped his Coke Zero with chunks of ice and we walked home arm in arm at about eleven. I read to Louis as I always do and he fell asleep around midnight, me too next to him with his book and my enlarging spectacles on my head.

In the cold morning I showered and gulped a few Panadol for breakfast and he packed his schoolbag and she shoved his Vegemite sandwiches and tangerines in his plastic blue favourite lunch box and she hurried off teaching and I drove my little boy to Christchurch Grammar School in leafy South Yarra.

As I drove by La Porcella Restaurant to get into Drummond Street we noticed the media outside it, lots of police and the sorts of plastic strip homicide tapes you see in TV police shows that indicate foul play and police helicopters buzzing overhead. I pulled up.

Lou was reading the lead story of *The Age*, which was about a murder that occurred the previous night inside La Porcella where Mick Gatto slew Andrew Veniamin over some dispute. Louis said as I got going, 'You know what Daddles? That Veniamin guy ought to have ordered takeaway.'

He is completely original to be with, the saving grace. A godsend, as my dad has said. He adores a no-fuss life. He hates bother. He loves me. Upon my fifty-ninth birthday he jumped down out of our doubledecker bunk and hugged me first thing, then jumped into my desk to draw me a funny cartoon birthday card with no prompting or expectation.

He's in Year 8 at high school and doing well. The other day he showed me a new essay his grade had to compose about keeping our beaches clean of trash; that was the moral within the fable he wrote in grey lead pencil with a few typos and cross-outs, with the opening line, 'Daddy looked evaporative.' No doubt he's a writer but he declares to me sometimes he won't for a living, having seen his father struggle.

Meantime at miserable Saint Michael's my son is finally on and playing singles in rotten conditions; you half expect a mammoth to roll the court. Fathers from Fitzroy Tennis Club are asleep and denied instant coffee to wake up. The lady who runs the club is pricking plastic sausages for the fatty sizzle and snarls at me for politely requesting a coffee, even though I am putting the electric kettle on. 'Just a minute, would you!'

Her face is contorted with loathing. She has a big backside and a love of control and I am right in her line of fire, but there is nowhere else to be. The Saint Michael's clubhouse is tiny with a sloping ping-pong table and ants everywhere in November. The Saint Michael's kids play our kids in doubles and the Saint Michael's kids' parents coach, which is against the rules but they do it anyway. The 'coaching' is barked ferociously from behind the cyclone-wire fence that separates their charges from their determination to win at any cost. I barrack wholeheartedly too for my son but never suggest this or that tactic, not like the Saint Michael's parents, who live only for victory. It is five degrees and people's eyes are watering with earliness and boredom and sleepy rage, due to pressure at work if they are fortunate enough to have any.

Although he is heading towards fourteen, my son is still like the child he was and sort of clings to his old father for human warmth in the atrocious veranda where we forlornly watch games going on; at the same time he wants to be independent and stands apart from me, and chastens me for sometimes being too glib or cynical in my muttered remarks, because my son is fair and gentle and honest.

I have always had trouble separating petty officialdom with reality and have always confused petty meanness with the absurdist poetry of Edward Lear, my idol. Lou is at last on, looking so laidback and just interested in playing at his level best, that is all really.

He warms up against a good Egyptian-born boy of the same young age, who is really very good, especially with a brilliant topspin rolled forehand that looks professional, a shot most handy in the unpredictable hurricane of perpetual Lalor. The background to the ugly courts is a tip.

Twigs of disagreeable, dirty broken branch flutter across the saturated fake grass tennis court where my son is rehearsing his serve. I am standing right by the Egyptian child's father who is coaching and yelling instructions so his son can win his match.

I am so cold I need to die. I get an old horse-blanket jumper from the boot; its neck is all scratchy but I keep it on to ward off the tempest. I can hear stricken sea lions.

It is a very close encounter but the other boy proves too good and my son goes up and shakes hands at the blowy net and then he wants a one-dollar sausage wrapped up in a thin envelope of plastic bread with imitation tomato sauce all through it. We play ping-pong with bats without handles. That was the only real fun we both had that day, the fun of the ping-pong after the Saint Michael's fathers finally wearied of playing and reluctantly gave us a go of it.

It felt good being a protective father at sixty at an unfriendly place like that. I turned forlornly back to Saint Michael's tennis courts and sat next to my adolescent boy. He was frozenly cheering on his team-mates and protested when I put a coat over his blue knees. Understandably I am a bit of a pain for all the fatherly fussing I do to him, but he is all I've got. He told me off in an undertone for fussing.

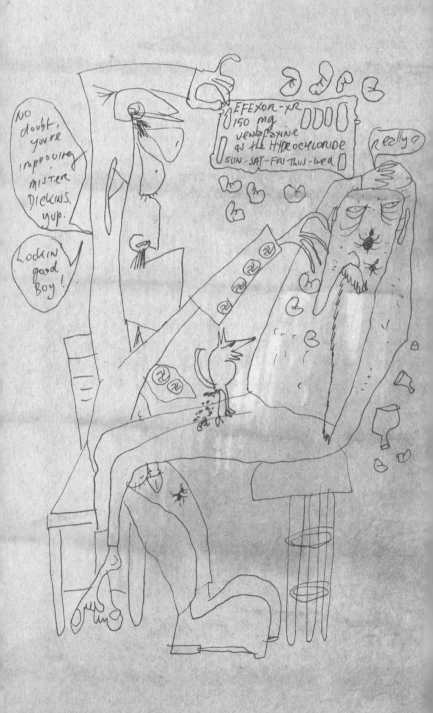

Chapter
five

THE CONUNDRUM OF being a single father is that due to admiration you are simultaneously a foe and a friend, but you must get your priorities right or you're nothing but an annoyance. When I do the pick-up after high school I am just like all the other fathers hanging around like vultures in the street. There is no parking and there is no work. We just hang around the street waiting. The other dads never say hi to me nor I to them. There is no rapport between us at all, and why should there be – we're Australian.

Their cars are better than mine, anyone's is. My car is just eighteen. It was born in Japan in 1990 and is rust-white in hue. It is filthy. I try hard as a single dad to keep it neat but tend to eat in it. Nuts go down the seat and create excoriating agony in your testicles or anus.

The air-conditioning unit doesn't work so well. The cold air is volcanic and accompanied by mire and dust. The heater freezes your body all along Punt Road. The right side wiper-rubber came off several times in New South Wales four years back and has never come back on.

Astonishingly my Corolla still goes. It does need a tune, but that's all. I'm just always in it. I may as well write in it. I am a chunky person but get into it easily, in fact in a second because the car is crucial to get my son to school, to get to the offices where various editors work who sometimes engage my services, to go to Luna Park with Louis and have a spin on the Big Dipper where life makes at last perfect sense.

A month back Louis bought himself a brand-new Wilson tennis bag at the deafening Epping Indoor Tennis Centre. I booked a court the evening before and we got there by 7 am on the Saturday, when he was rostered off in his tennis 'comp'. The explosion of the acoustics was sensational. Although a bit slow, I hit some strong first serves in against him poised like a whippet up the other end, scampering around like a will-o'-the-wisp. He is gifted and we play all the time, so my next wife will have to be keen on tennis.

Although it's hard to look after oneself after separation, it is the tennis between my son and me that gives us both a lift in spirits. I know throughout this book I have satirised and heaped scorn on the hospital, where I suffered so much as well as got overdue help; I am grateful to the nurses for putting maximum pressure on me to shower first thing in the morning, shampoo my hair and eat my breakfast. I still can't believe I went back to my bed in the middle of the afternoon. It had to be boredom or more depression, surely, or both.

All the prescription drug packets that did me no good at all are scattered in my rented pharmaceutical cupboard along with the Gold Brand hay fever eyedrops and amicable Gold Brand cotton buds to try to dig the wax out of my ears, not that I always want to catch what strangers are saying. I like being a monk.

I want to write about last Sunday now as it sits upon me and revisits – rechronicles itself in my storytelling self. It was not so hot as the day that forty-seven degrees was achieved and hundreds of my fellow Victorians died in the bushfires: the most unimaginable death I can think of apart from working as a poet in Australia.

I packed up Louis's things and my tennis stuff and zipped up his still new-looking Wilson tennis bag, which has pouches for our two racquets and room too for the five bucks I am charged at the Clifton Hill Courts to hit the ball with my young boy who plays 'comp' there every Saturday at exactly 7 am. We're both boys.

It was muggy and I was hung over – I had polished off nearly two bottles of off-shore chardonnay and smoked half a packet and sat relaxed with two fans on my body watching some boring rubbish on television the night before – and we got in the car and my palms were singed by the insufferable heat of the plastic steering wheel and burning-hot plastic grey gearshift as soon as we both hopped in. I confessed I used intemperate language and Louis looked shocked as mostly I do not. I try not to swear at all and detest it in others but it seems perfectly understandable when I stoop to it. Anyway he was shocked when Daddy swore due to heat mixed with bad hangover.

I drove okay to the Clifton Hill courts right on Hoddle Street, where there is always the most eye-watering stink that emanates from a big and burst excrement pipe, which gave out due to stress long ago because people in Clifton Hill seem to shit too much. I felt like a hyperventilating pensioner and pack mule the way I had all our stuff under my arms, and I plonked the tennis bag down and Louis innocently fumbled a giant in-the-fridge-all-night plastic bottle of Lo-Cal lemonade and I had a go at him and like a sudden viper I hissed at him, 'Dumb!'

All the healthy, natural, freckled colour fled from his handsome face because Daddy had cursed him. In his fourteen years of existence I had never mocked him, not once no matter how I wanted to say something when he had broken something I valued such as a thirty-nine-buck Japanese electric fan he trod on as soon as he came into my hovel after the school pick-up one hot afternoon. He sheared the plastic propeller shaft in two, in one fell swoop. I was shattered. I'd just bought it and now it was useless and the rental house was like an oven.

At the Clifton Hill tennis courts when I said 'Dumb!', like a gander going by the pulverised expression in that fair face I have kissed and adored since he was born fourteen years ago – that look was the look of a very sensitive boy. More like a young man.

He stared at his birth father in an entirely new way in that rare second of hate that I felt for his clumsiness but it was my fault of course for being hung over (I'm hung over once a week) and anyway he was devastated and stood unafraid right up to me and whispered right through me into my memory and my immortal fathering soul with purest righteous indignation, stock-still is how he stood and squared-off at me: 'You called me dumb.' His look withered me and aged me and it assassinated me with its pinpoint accuracy of meaning and portent.

'Well, not exactly you, Louis,' I stumbled and gulped somewhat, trying to look away from the accusations in both his blue pure eyes. He packed up his Wilson tennis bag with an assertive zip and wheeled round to get going. He wanted out of there. But I said, 'Look, Lou, I'm so sorry, I shouldn't have called you dumb because that is obviously incorrect, in fact it's obviously an insult and as a consequence I am shattered to think I have criticised you when all you did, in fact, was to fumble a king-sized bottle of chilled Lo-Cal lemonade in the dust but it didn't burst so we can still have a slug of it, old bean.' I have always called Louis 'Old Bean'. He calls me 'Old Cheese' and refers to himself on the tennis court as 'Young Cheese'.

We went on and played but he wouldn't congratulate Old Cheese on any of his rare winners, though I did his many swift winners; I praise them as he is really good and that day hit the racquet out of my hand with a 120 kph two-handed backhand-drive delivered right at my member (if I still have one between my legs; I'll have to check next when I'm in the shower).

He was cold and unforgiving and it was a bad match between a sensitive and idealistic adolescent who is nimble and zestful compared to his saggy-eyed father who loves him whatever incarnation of him it is. He seems to be growing longer limbs as I write this to him. He is the only person who loves me. My father called him a godsend. He is but I must not lean on him. It's difficult not to as he's the closest soul to me.

Eventually after a wrecked set I sat down near the Clifton Hill public loo – the one that is perennially padlocked – why do tennis clubs love to padlock their Porta-Loos? I usually hang on if I am dying to urinate as they love to lock their entire clubhouse too. I began to speak to him about being lonely after living with his mother since 1982 but he did not understand my grief and was still out with me over the stupid 'dumb' insult of ninety minutes earlier. The stupidest moment of my life that was. How could I have insulted an angel on earth? He's the one I'm constantly drawing. He's the perfect host. I'm his friend, I hope, and not his adviser, his dumb coach, his foolish sage who wouldn't have a clue how to father.

I said I didn't blame his mother but I was lonely and I shouldn't have said that because you have to be a role model and suppress all weakness because you only burden a child. He cried too and said it was hard for him at school because all the kids realised he comes from a broken home. He put his elongating strong limbs round my Charles-Laughton gargoyle visage and shuddered with me while contented families bounded round the artificial grass, having a ball with the unminding fluorescent ball that comes in a can if you've got ten bucks. Usually we have an ice-cream after a hit but he didn't want one. He slumped in the suffocating car on the awful way home to my place. I said would you like to take a shower but he said the towels were filthy and that is quite right, Lou, they all are. I don't know how to live. I am as domesticated as an ape. No wonder the marriage fell through.

He is her in all his limbs, and all his witty ways are the wit I fell in love with and was the lover of for nearly three decades. He jokes a bit like her, throwaway one-liners, and is full of life like her and those incredible English, so English, sulks, can last weeks! You are lying down on nails for them to step over and they still decline to relent. Pack your stuff.

On Christmas morning she was in her renovated home and looked great with no need of elbow-crutch or sympathy. I asked her whether or not she was experiencing any pain but she said she felt terrific and she looked that way as well. She made our son and me a delicious breakfast of fried eggs and crispy bacon on toast. She gave me a whole jug of percolated coffee. I purred. We exchanged gifts and our son was happy as we did so, making lots of tiny word plays he grew up with, household words, word associations, routines and comical capers on the spot, which he excels at and he in fact is the funniest fellow in our tiny broken family trying to be whole again; not easy, is it.

The sources of strength are my grandmother and my father.
It is their will that I inherited and their staying power.
They *will* live.

Luckily for me I can write and draw and so defeat temporarily the awful sensations of uselessness and pointlessness of life alone. Since the break-up I can't cook; no matter what I do I spill it and burn it and can't fry an egg properly. All toast burns bright and dull black to a cinder. My instant coffee is the only thing I don't muck up. I drink it by the weir to wake up after long drugless repose.

My wife just rang me to say her car was burnt out the front by junkies and she can't get insurance because it's in my name;

the cops, she said, were very rude to her. The cop who found the burnt-out car berated her. The same old life, the same old pressures. When I beheld her in hospital recently, it softened the rancour in my heart to see her in a hospital bed with rehab looming and her hip sort of fixed up. It is very much a disconnecting life and a strange way to relate to someone, but you soldier on notwithstanding or not with sitting.

I've been advised to brighten this opus up but I think the general reader will find solace in its truth, not its jokes or exaggerations. Everything I say is an exaggeration to make an impact. I can't be lived with or for or anything remotely like marriage. My wife did the only thing she could possibly do with me and that was to leave me.

I don't resent her for that decision. She suffered for twenty-seven years as a result of my comic-hysteria. I'm a practising hysteric borne out of my mother's comic womb. The other night my wife was on the phone but I wasn't listening. I was rather more giving full attention to the bottom bit of the doubledecker bed my son and I repose in from time to time. The room's a wreck and I can't be bothered tidying it up. I stared at my pillow and again realised no one but my body was to join me. No one but my Quasimodo ugliness fits it. My unfit body with aches all in it. Lying there in state, just about. At least I'm not drugged. But as she spoke in her amicable manner late at night I knew she was only contented because Louis was with her at her place.

The hardest thing is the innocence of your little boy. Who understands that it is over and final. That he stays with Mummy during the week and Daddy the weekend. But he says, 'Which house are we doing the tree at this Christmas?' Or else, 'Where shall we all celebrate my fourteenth birthday?'

Louis ennobles the meanest of things merely by being next to them and then all you see are flowers. He makes flowers of words and bouquets of snapshots. Even the way he chews his food is noble. Modest and innocent and pleasant and trusting. I'm transported with him. Flying first-class all the way.

Nothing aches when he is near. We play basketball each morning; he loudly echoes his bright orange basketball right next to his father's writing-desk, in the little home office; in the skinny doorway he bounces and his grin bounces and he implores, 'Come along, Old Cheese, let's do a few hoops, eh?' So we stroll, talking and joking, up to the local park and I commence proceedings with a corner-ball, which is difficult. A corner ball requires the thrower to pitch the basketball twenty metres and you need quite an arm on you to do it. His eyes say, 'Come on, Daddy, you can do it!' I nearly got one this morning; it hit the steel rim, a close thing.

The thing about children playing is that they tire of sentences in the end, no matter how clever they are; they are sick of talk and they need to hurl something, to chuck a ball at a ring.

I make a mental note never to be too tired for my son. He bounds around like a leaf or a jaybird and his weight's a fraction of mine but children must play.

Our friend, the just-pumped-up basketball, accompanies us through uneven, bluestone, winding, old North Carlton lanes until we see if the gates of Lee Street Primary School are unpadlocked; one usually is, so we in cloud and sunshine bounce our ball along until we arrive at the park. We ignore the trendies with their fashionable baby-strollers and correct-thinking eunuch fathers and throw the basketball into energetic immediate life that never ends in any way. Joy doesn't. It just goes on and on, like laughter.

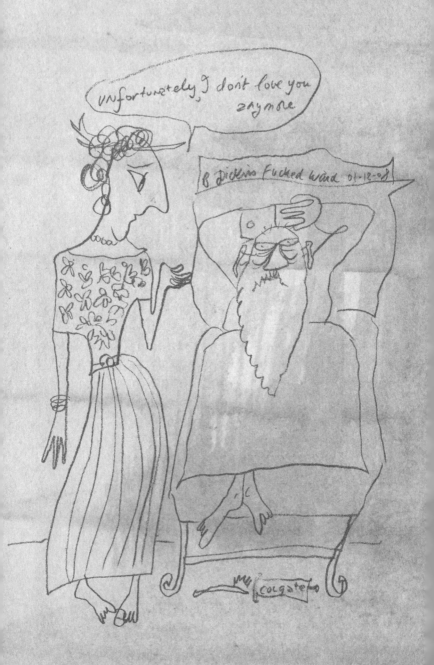

Chapter
six

WHEN ONE SPLITS UP one's friends magnify somehow and are shot through with divinity. Two days ago it was quite hot and it was a lonely sort of a Sunday, and I didn't really feel like writing or drawing or being alone; my mind was wanting company. I rang my filmmaker friend Brian McKenzie and he invited me over to their home in leafy Kew for a sausage. I felt just like one so I went over there, feeling sleepy as it had been a bad night with lots of tossing and turning and so on. I was lonely.

Their daughter Sophie showed me a really good new lead-pencil drawing of figs that put me in mind of the very best of Brett Whitely's pencil drawings, a great looseness and grandeur of infinitesimal detail. She did a portrait of me once in oils and in it I look like a Neanderthal, which is in part what I am. I've always felt like a cave person. When having a sausage with my friends the McKenzies, everything I saw there seemed like writing or drawing, and I was having difficulty separating real existence with books or theatre. Is life art? No, it is certainly nothing like it, I think you'll find.

Liz McKenzie saw I was rubbing my wrists and forearms a bit as we chatted in their garden, next thing she gave me some sort of arthritis ointment she has been employing for her own comfort, and her husband's, who suffers from all sorts of aches and nerve pain. She said to me in the garden, 'Why don't you keep this and use it at your home?'

I couldn't help but think of how preoccupied I was at my rental property much of the time; on the way up their street I stopped in awe of the sheer magnificence of the huge mansions covered in autumnal gardeners and nannies for the pampered children of the Kew Nouveau Riche and I thought of how hemmed in I was whenever I was working, with no room to swing a cat. I'm always knocking things over due to crampedness. It isn't that the McKenzies are rich and comfortable with so many bedrooms and a big garden that is perhaps small as far as Kew gardens go, but that my courtyard is so small I go into it and disappear. I can't do anything but sit.

One of their daughters, Grace, is off to India next Sunday; and I asked her how she was feeling about going there, to which she replied, 'Oh, not too bad, I suppose.' The only romantic destination I send my son to is Safeway in Drummond Street, Carlton, where we search hard for Nutri-Grain and a bottle of fresh milk. That's our holiday. Going nowhere.

Writing and drawing are my best loves, my colleagues, and I know they would never let me down, not like some people, but you mustn't be vindictive. Everyone does their level best. It's just that some of them levelled me.

I swore at an old friend on the phone today; that was stupid of me. He had upset me in his comfortable, paid-off home in Clifton Hill. He bullshitted around with his artistic soup and sipped stubbies and raved on about the cutting-edge balsa-wood gliders he designs and flies, and where he goes for a walk to fill in his day. Everything I said he contradicted. I just wished he'd blow away like a cumulonimbus; his superiority and boredom with me, the way he looked down when I tried to storytell so that lack of eye-contact stuffed things up, and he knew it. He wore me to the veritable stump. I told him, 'I'm going through separation and all you care about is your stupid soup and your ice-cold stubbies!' I should have added something like take a good look for your heart, why not? It might be under the bed, then you can put it on.

I had a very restless night indeed, with a friend, a good one, a writer like me, ringing me late at night when I was writing this. He was upset and high – exciting to talk to but it was just too late to be ringing; as a result I didn't get a wink. It is quite tough being a writer in a country that doesn't seem to have any need of them.

Why are comfortable people cruel? It's indifference. You embarrass them by being lonely. I drank wine yesterday and chainsmoked to conquer nothing; as nothing is wrong with me to begin with. It's just a habit. It has taken twenty-three hours to get sober with nausea, headache and guilt. Dear old guilt.

Peter Luby, the screenwriter and wit, dropped over at six last night and he cooked some delicate casserole that I dropped straight down my favourite shirt. We raved until he left, then I collapsed in my lonely bunk and before unconsciousness arrived I had the foresight to switch the big electric fan on. Unluckily for me it has come off its metal stem with a tormented screw so the only way I can cool my body down in the cramped house is to carry the thing around with me. I have now decided to go sober and smoke-free for the remainder of my life because both of those terrible drugs are doing me no good at all.

Drinks don't make the marriage come back. It's an oscillating time for the author of this life at the moment of destruction and creation; naught can be done to resurrect my past that had so much happiness and escapism in it. I realise that and understand that punishment equals enlightenment through suffering. Yesterday one wept all of the day. And discovered only very sore eyes.

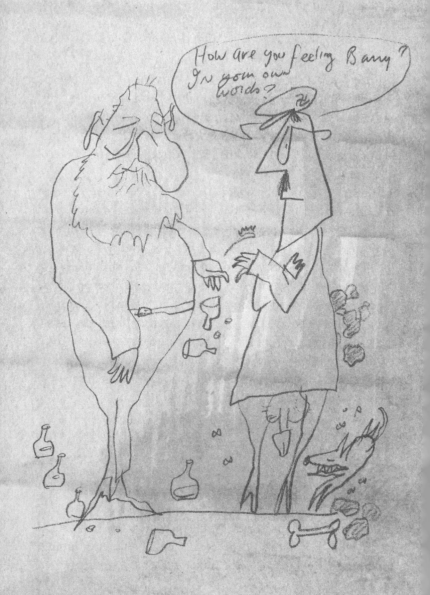

Chapter
seven

WITH HIS FRIENDLINESS my son is a special guest at my place, just the fun of his company I find so enchanting. He likes me to read to him at night; we usually retire around eleven-thirty on the Saturday or Sunday, after a spot of television; he tends to channel-surf which leaves me unable to keep up, then he undresses with me out of the bedroom. It's so touching to be a loving daddy to a small and trusting growing-up boy of almost fourteen, limbs elongating as in some sort of Modigliani drawing in charcoal.

He sleeps tranquilly when he's with me. I love to watch him set up an aerodrome-lamp-thing my determined father gave me so I could read his nightly pages. It is blinding and my old eyes water when he switches the stupid thing on me. The other evening he placed a sheet of folded newspaper over its big bulb with a saucepan sheath-object around it so it would be 'less bright'. It wasn't less bright and my eyes watered like a river.

I read eleven or so pages of Jeremy Clarkson's latest collection of essays and he chuckled at the cleverness in the writing; he enjoys good writing and is a nifty author himself, as it transpires, and got ninety-three in the last term of his high school for English Expression, which is precisely as it ought to be.

He is so cool in his manner and warm to me without effort; he isn't sentimental but liberated.

People who read me in the papers say, 'Where do you get all your ideas from?' I take from this my ideas of comedy and terror. I think they come from ordinary life then I magnify them for effect to amuse or enrage the reader. Two weeks ago my son and I went to the countryside to see Ross Luscombe and his boy named Boyd. The plan was to get to Castlemaine and have a belt of the tennis ball on the courts. I haven't done much country driving since I got out of the hospital; all my driving has been achieved in the city's usual surreal franticness. I'm a good driver but was a bit apprehensive about hoons and demon truckdrivers. Louis keeps all of our tennis stuff in his Wilson tennis carry-all. We got hold of our shirts and shorts and I parked a bottle of water in the Corolla in case it got hot. I filled the tank and got on the Calder Freeway. You bear right just past the old Essendon Airport, which has been not there for forty years.

I live entirely in the past, and my sense of locations has to do with the 1950s and 1960s; I do try to keep up with modern architecture and contemporary freeways, but there's not much I can do about ugliness and density of traffic – what my friend Jim Davidson calls 'hoonage', meaning the exact measurement of morons per hectare. In short I don't fit.

I drove to the Bendigo turn-off and swung to the right to follow the road to Castlemaine, and it came to me that it wasn't so hard to keep up with my fellow motorist or rockmelon deliverer. We sipped the cold bottled water and chewed some still-cold Kit Kats to keep up our energy levels and got in one piece to Castlemaine.

I parked in Lyttleton Street, rang Ross on the mobile, so he and son Boyd appeared and we headed for the tennis courts at Castlemaine, which I remembered being of gorgeous green natural edible grass. Instead they were made from indestructible rubber and bizarre bitumen. Horrid. We played for ninety minutes and switched sides so that Boyd became my partner and Lou played with Ross. It was fun and both Louis and Boyd played really great, though Ross was the twinkletoes. He has an uncanny style with spin and applied so much spin on the Head tennis ball that it just about came back over the net. We laughed and enjoyed the exercise. As in an Escher engraving, the vortex of surreal tennis courts went on forevermore. There had to have been forty empty courts with no sound nor movement upon any of them. We were the only players.

After a few matches we shared a chocolate thickshake at a place called Trogg. Ross wanted to show off his farm at Muckleford, about twenty minutes away, and that was pleasant too. He showed me his new chocolate-coloured lounge room carpet and comfortable easy chairs, and the view of the countryside was uplifting and relaxing. He is a great gardener and I enjoyed inspecting his lettuces.

His son Boyd wanted Louis to 'do a sleep-over'; we both wanted to, but also wanted to get home to the city, so we reluctantly waved farewell to them and I drove back on the Calder Freeway, so nuclear and different from the highway I used to know. Brave New Freeway. I felt vulnerable in my old worn-out car. In short I was afraid.

It was overcast and I was slightly perspiring in the cabin of the 1990 Corolla I go everywhere in. Lou was playing peacefully with his Playstation, the one I helped pay for at Christmas, and I was aware of the speed the other drivers were travelling at. Over the 110 kph-limit and giving me the finger for being too slow. A gigantic truck flew in from my left on a feeder into the freeway and because it was now raining hard the windscreen was saturated. I had the wipers on high and the weather changed alarmingly and spontaneously, as it does in Victoria near Christmas. It was a hail and rain tempest. I could barely see due to the storm, and the mosquitoes biting into my ear canals made it quite trying, I have to say. Louis contentedly played with his new Christmas present and nibbled a mint oblivious to my latest calamity.

Strive as I might I couldn't steer that well or see anything but blurry scarlet and cadmium orange brake and tail-lights of trucks and cars all going over the limit in their rush to arrive back in town, sixty kilometres away from where Lou and I were at the sodden moment. The demister didn't work and the interior of the car was completely fogged. I was alarmed at the fogginess within the car and for once wished I had the income to purchase a new car and not put my child's life and my life at risk due to artistic poorness. I swore.

The ramming-speed trucks, abrim with iceberg fresh Safeway lettuce and billiard-ball baby tomatoes and nuclear carrots, just kept coming through the rained-away freeway and the cars around me aquaplaned and the whole thing ended up terrifying. Louis kept playing with his Playstation and I kept on swearing with genuine fear, which was justifiable given the quirky circumstances.

My old heart she pounded and I tried to keep my cool as the inevitability of worry caused anxieties to re-weave in my tired body; I'd felt too tired to drive to Muckleford from Castlemaine but as I love Ross I did it, and struggled with the worry again, unsure as to either pull over and wait for it to stop or just grit my dentures and keep driving to Melbourne. At least it didn't stall. That would have been the end. But it didn't.

I had to pull over so I flipped on the left indicator and got well over to let the giant trucks steam by in their violent manner; so many of them way over the speed-limit. I felt like town mouse out of his humble zone and clashing with titans of frozen groceries heading for a billion customers. A Sudanese taxi driver gave me the finger and mocked me in his own language.

I waited twenty-five minutes by the side of the Calder Highway and then the roof of our car was struck deafeningly by thousands upon thousands of table-tennis-sized hailstones so I couldn't hear what my little boy was saying, not that he was anxious. I was terrified. Why didn't my mechanic fix the wipers, as he said he would?

Over the course of the past twenty years working as a writer I've averaged $40,000–$50,000 and can't afford such items as a new car or what aren't really luxuries at all but seem it, such as good new clothes. I'm broke. Nearly all Australian authors are. It's how it is here.

As I sat in hailstony silence inside the car I remembered all the disagreements with my wife, and that many of them had to do with money. The pressure contributing to my share of things like mortgage payments, power accounts, gas bills, car registration and all the demanding myriad bills. The appalling hailstones quit as smartly as they arrived and so I pulled, politely using the right indicator, into traffic again.

To my dismay the right windscreen wiper became lodged on the far right rubber of the front windscreen itself and declined obstinately to spring back to the centre of the screen to recommence its squeegee action so necessary during storms.

I couldn't see a thing. Then it recommenced hailing like many Gestapo boots reverberating on the thin tin ceiling of my vehicle.

I apologised to my son for swearing but he said in his stoic way, 'That's okay, Daddy.' I got to the next town and drove into a garage just so I could hear myself think; I got under some cover and put in twenty bucks' worth of unleaded just to make sure we were both okay to make it to Melbourne. I bought my son some potato chips. I got home okay and we watched some silly show on television. I had a hot shower and wound down from watching anything that moved. I would have laughed at a gas account.

After the hurly-burly of that bad ride home it felt luxurious to see my son in his T-shirt and warm snug pyjamas lazily reading a comic in his top part of the doubledecker bed in my new home. He fell asleep while I read to him from his new favourite book by Jeremy Clarkson.

When I read to my son aloud from the selection of mordant literature dripping from the plume of a man who can really write, like Jeremy Clarkson, it felt as if there were no chasm at all between wealthy authors and strugglers.

Louis is buoyant and floats like a cork; he is never upset and hates 'bother' and he abhors what he calls 'bogans', those rough types who swear all the time and drink themselves too stupid to be good fellows. There are only two intellectuals in Australia: myself and you who read me.

My father read aloud to John and me in the old bungalow; it was the assurance given by the reader to his snoozy children – the promise that literature is for you. Literature was loved by he who gave me an instant trust for it; a profound respect. How different from my trendy bald psychiatrist who boasted to an English teacher that he never reads.

My English tutor was my father. He read his memory off. He always had a book between his inky and honest fingers. He never once smudged a single snow-white page out of rushing or absent-mindedness. He built his own library and used to attend the Melbourne University Book Fair. Home with a kitbag full of classics like *Moby Dick* and *The Old Curiosity Shop* and *The Practical Handyman's Guide to Things to Do and Make*.

Later on my English teacher became my first wife, Sarah, whose effortless dialogue was like meeting Oscar Wilde. She spoke as well as she wrote and her household repartee was showbusiness, a phenomenon she caught from her mother

Margaret, who was always being brilliant all over the place. She called one of her favourite authors, 'My delicious Graeme Greene!' You can't top that for intimacy.

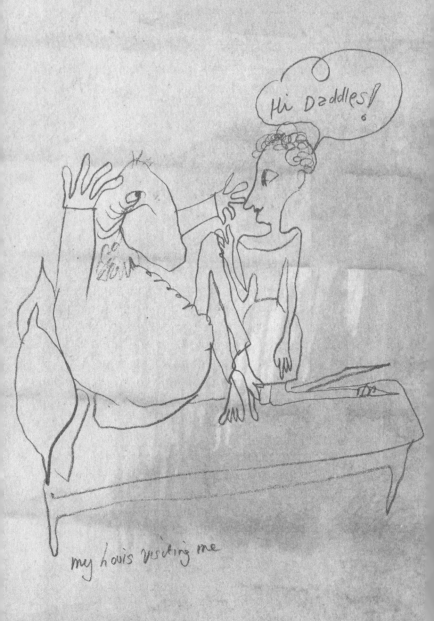

Chapter
eight

I BOUGHT AN INFLATABLE DINGHY last week for $45 with black
screwable oars and a foot pump for my son. We laughed just
pumping it up and like contented mammals we knelt to sniff
the brand newness that proffered fun and guaranteed giggles.
I bought it at Whittlesea and drove up that way just to be
nearer trees. Louis laughed and we inspected the emergency
puncture kit in case it struck a rock somehow; we pumped it
up in my miniature kitchen and smiled at the oblong boat the
bright bit of plastic or rubber once was in its new kit. Louis
eagerly screwed the plastic oars together and I boiled the kettle
to manufacture myself a cup of coffee to try to wake.

I tethered the inflated dinghy on the roof of my faithful
Corolla and we motored to Middle Park last Saturday morning
at eight in the not-awake-yet-gorgeous daylight. I was so
sleepy I forgot where Middle Park was. I found it in the end
because it's the ocean. A herd of middle-aged cyclists looking
just like the Third Reich were puffing and panting, all bunched
with bottoms up and pursed lips and clenched lips along The
Esplanade where the beach is. One of them, my age, swore at
me for driving an offensive vehicle.

I examined the parking signs and made out all the rules

making parking a jail term. It was a clearway until 10.30 am. So instead I drove to Sandringham Yachting Club, where men my age still wear waxed handle-barred twirled moustaches and use the word 'nigger'.

I was astonished to read on the parking machine it cost five bucks per hour to park your Corolla there, even though it was a very mild and pleasant Saturday morning. I tipped my ashtray out for what men of my generation call 'shrapnel' and inserted seven dollars forty in ten-cent coins and we untied the dinghy and carried it and the wonderful oars to the foreshore.

The water was gentler and crystalline and I couldn't make out a shark or poisonous jellyfish so we went in, my son over-excitedly jumping in it and getting at the screw-together-oars, and we both made the same joke at the same time of 'heading for Tasmania'. My old chest was stiff with glee and I felt young again. My young son sure grinned straight in my eyes and he sparkled as he said, 'Gee, Dad, this is the best holiday I've had this year!' And he hadn't got one this year. The few minutes or playful hours we spent mucking about in the seawater made him say that. The entire length of hot January he spent at his homes: his mother's house and my rental property.

It was beautiful to motor down to the Sandringham Royal Yachting Club together – it was the only place I could possibly think of – and pay for the outrageous public parking, grumbler in thongs and old father, on a Sunday when my son was desperate to play (all children must, and all parents must) and then to both tiptoe up to disentangle the little bit of tricky white greasy string I kept in the back of the faithful white Corolla and let loose the inflatable dinghy.

He was enraptured as he grasped the assemble-yourself, black plastic oars and commenced rowing operations. The waves were friendly, everything was. A whole lot of fitness freaks were inflating their expensive bicycles for an assertive whiz through the ti-tree but we didn't care much about their importance, my son and I. We were out for a sail.

Louis laughed at the sight of our boat bumping about in the splashy clean beach water; I trod with due care on the dark and gritty ocean sand as I didn't need to cut my feet on any razor-sharp stones or Man-of-War creatures. I have an ingrown fear of sharp things, especially words.

He called out to me in sheerest joy, 'Come on, Daddy, your turn of the new inflatable boat! Come on, Daddy! You get in too with me, Daddy!' I tried to but only got one right knee into it then tipped backwards as I went in the drink; the icy delicious water instantly giving me relief from the heat. I shivered impressively.

Though tired and fraught I always rally to the call of playing. When I was still married, Louis and I hit the ball along the concrete and eroded tar paths that in their remarkably friendly fashion wound through that childish park near our home of ten years in Canning Street. He caught the tram home from Christchurch Grammar School and had a cold drink and a quick wash of the hot young eager face and we chipped and volleyed. The stragglers home from dreary office jobs sometimes glanced at us as though to think, 'Look at that old fool hit the ball with the nice neat schoolboy!'

We used to hit one shot really hard heavenwards with the old fluffless ball sailing up like the soul of someone who'd that second died. We called that particular stroke 'A heaven shot' and Louis used to point at its instant height and instant descent. 'Do it again, Daddy! The heaven shot again!'

When I read to him – at the minute it is Lemony Snicket and he enjoys the style – he is like perfect rapture in a quiet contemplative way and there is no vanity or arrogance in him but the same stillness and trust and acceptance he had at the point of birth and delivery into an uncertain world.

My wife and I used once to read to each other in our bed bought by me at Myers. She would lean on my shoulder and fall asleep as I read to her from her best books and she'd gently murmur and almost paraphrase those astonishing sentences she'd memorised as a girl from Emily and Charlotte Brontë. I got so many of the nuances wrong but she forgave me by correcting me. What I'd truly give to try to read those sentences aloud to her. I read them to myself to pacify myself.

I understand why men kill themselves after they are separated. I'll not. I have a son I love much more than me. With him I have a rapport and he is cleverer than me, like everyone else I meet in the street these days. He's a riot really, but a detached and rare one, at least, as he detests fuss. He said that to me one night in my home, lying in peace on the above bunk with his elongating limbs so relaxed and his hands clasped on his bosom looking up at the cheap dark, 'Daddy, I hate fuss.'

Then he fell asleep and I gave him his Weet-Bix and honey in the morning with chilled fresh milk. He did his homework and I tidied the place by casting saturated bath mats out over the back lane where they made an agreeable sound in the filth donated by neighbours who live as hogs. We're all cave chaps after all. But I cut his Nutella white bread sandwiches and installed a large chilled Kit Kat in his blue plastic clip-on-lunchbox. God, you should see how many books he puts in his heavy schoolbag!

The morning is order. It is Louis's fresh sandwiches and a nice big fresh banana and a little bag of crisps as he has a good appetite lately. I drop over to my former home and feel tortured in a way because of all my wife's portraits hanging on her walls and all the furniture we bought together and paintings given to me. I can't get myself to go there.

Human loneliness and despair are my oldest paramours. I have always adored them both where everything else is false and not worth the effort of bothering about. I told my wife on the telephone tonight I wanted a divorce and that would make a clean break and possibly we can meet someone new to love us. She replied it was no use talking about it on the phone but to arrange a date to discuss it. It was so hot in my bedroom and writing room and I had a small electric fan as per usual aimed right at my face. I cried harder than charity. I walked up to the local park after translating my useless hurt to bitter tears, born out of a deep well of emptiness and stupefaction. It is not hate but the emptiness of my spirit that is burying me but each morning I am so disciplined and shower at five and sip instant coffee in the small courtyard where the air can be cool before it heats up to the full horror.

The hectic traffic in Carlton gets me confused and I am careful and assertive as I can be as I weave our way between gay and lesbian cyclists, all of whom ignore me. They all give me the finger and cycle so assertively I want to give up driving because I, Barry Dickins, am destroying the Ozone Layer. I am personally responsible for global warming. Everything is my fault as is well chronicled.

Louis didn't sleep well the night before last and looked droopy on our way to his high school. I showed him his banana and big bottle of chilled orange soft drink, the kind that all good athletes swear by, Crimson Gatorade and his chilled giant chunky Kit Kat chocolate bar and he said, 'Thank you, Daddy.' He enjoys modern history and on our way to school sometimes asks me who this or that famed citizen was or is. He bowerbirds facts away and so do I, except I remember things the way I want rather than the dreary way they actually are.

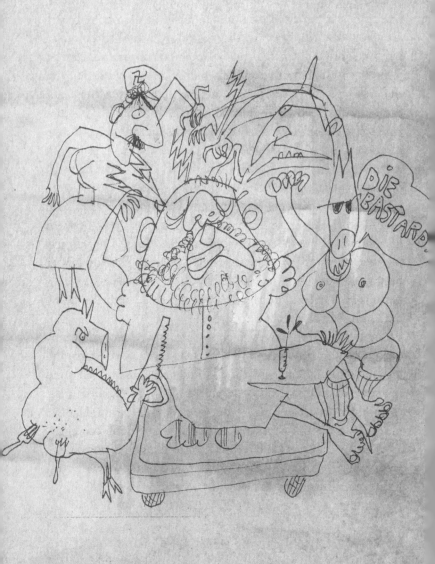

Chapter
nine

I TRY TO GET to my old home on Sundays to see how my parents are. Cooking and cleaning are difficult as my old father has bad rheumatoid arthritis in his back and even in his fizzy fingertips and shows me the way of them, pantomiming their uselessness the very second I get inside their dwelling. It's the thespian in him. Where I got it from. The instantaneous theatre of the absurd. He's an absurdist like me.

'I could hardly stand up in the spa,' he sorrowed and told me how bad his feet were in graphic detail so that I felt ill with worry, sleepless.

I asked him if he was going to turn the spa on, pointing out that it was forty-two degrees that day, and that his concrete patio's heat was the equal of the surface of the sun, no doubt of it.

'Your mother gets distressed by the sound it makes,' he complained with a roll of the eyes to show the irony. Everything he is comes from irony and sarcasm except for when he's a patriot. He's a war hero. A modest one.

'Gee, Dad, that's a shame she gets upset by the chugging action of a spa filling up. So does that also mean she won't get in for a cool-off?' I knew the answer before I asked the question but asked it anyway just to get in the groove of his home. He's been in it since 1945, when his dad built it.

Of her ongoing mental illness he once declared, 'I married her in sickness and in health. She leaves here over my dead body.' Point made, father.

It's unimaginable he should die and not be there, my honest father, impossible as the deep-fried tomatoes beyond withering on their crucifixion stakes in his heat-shimmer garden. Though plagued by back pain and stiffness in both worn-out knees and fizzy feelings in fingertips so he cannot get a grip on objects and swears beneath his breath lest he fumbles something – he's always had a sure grip – he just grates his false teeth and does another long day.

When my mother comes out of her unusual mental condition – never seeing anyone or lifting a finger to help cook or clean – she brings photosynthesis over to her side and her feet need to dance again, possibly with him, and in short she cheers up.

I can find no fault with my old family because I'm such a sinner myself who has forfeited his marriage because of slovenliness. My new rental property became a slum as soon as I turned the key. It is filthy as a fit. I try to clean it, half-heartedly.

Another recent Sunday I was invited to a farewell party for a woman I was lovers with in 1972 and we briefly dwelt in a cave. Her name is Gwenda and I hadn't seen her since the cave in Stawell. We lived as Adam and Eve in a rock dwelling situated in the Grampians, which another girl I went to school with, Nereda Dunkly, had shown me. Those relaxing cave days came back in a single second as I looked at her through so many decades. Her bloke met her through me; he was Sid Clayton, a bohemian and talented postman I met in Carlton in 1970 in Lygon Street bopping along replete in a drip-dry, sky-blue postman's shirt complete with tin whistle and letter sack on his brawny shoulders. I loved him as soon as I saw him because he was so laidback.

She was called 'Gwen Indian' and in our fabled cave she painted her breasts with spirals of my oil paint; I remember she enjoyed doing that in the front sitting room of our cave. We lived on campfire burnt toast and incredible views. My mother took out a missing persons advertisement in the *Sun News Pictorial* and Gwen and I read it with interest in the cave. I looked better in the picture in the paper than I did in real life. I remember during our ten-day stint in the cave I once broke off a grey, dehydrated, hollow tree branch just like in *Tarzan of the Apes* and got an impressive fire going and chased what I thought was a hare. Gwenda was a great lover and she never ever tired.

That is a long time ago and a billion depressions and boredoms, births, deaths and excitements have occurred since the cave, but it was a good sensation to see her again at her party as she prepared to return to Canada. Her daughter Bella just had a baby and today for the first time in thirteen years I held a real live baby in my arms. I felt redeemed and realised what rot goes through my mish-mashed mind.

I didn't consume any alcohol nor smoke and for the past few weeks have gone clear, understanding I have to be in good health to drive my son to high school as well as to write and draw all day without fogginess. Drink just mucks me up.

One of the aspects of aloneness that is unbearable is never to be touched. The intimacy of being touched is almost beyond my remembrance these days as I go to bed alone and always sleep, dream and nightmare alone, never being kissed by anybody else and listening to one's breath in the doubledecker. To be willingly kissed and caressed and kidded and made love to without ever tiring is what I am after each day without success.

I miss the days when my paternal grandmother looked after

me in Sydney when I was eleven – she displayed the mythic streets to me and the fantasy steam and electric trains of Sydney Central Railway Station and accompanied me to her sister Nelly's place like a sherpa up the hills and hot winding backblocks of Cronulla where I slept in a hut with Uncle Ted, who was Nell's lover, no doubt of that.

Even the way she spoke to me: it was patient and considered and her voice was my voice only exactly sixty years older and her true voice was a girl's one that was stoical and strong and sure of its history. She was real working class, like I happen to be. Someone born where no writers go to term. My grandmother was funny the way my son Louis is: effortless and untutored and beyond influence. They would have got on had she lived more than a hundred.

I miss such things as my older brother John and I going to see *Lawrence of Arabia* at the pictures that once were in town that we all called Melbourne. Being able to dawdle and chat and have a chewie on the train with all its suffocating windows slid up to snare the merest asthma attack of cool change. To comb our hair together in our family tiny bathroom in a skerrick of mirror and look good to go out together and never have a clue what he was to say, or me. Just mates.

My mother flipping over two-inch-thick pancakes stuffed with apple and heavenly coagulant sugar in her warped iron frying pan and her honest pre-sickness noble forehead dripping with sweat and standing by with athletic arms and kind big smile and the radio on and playing the Beatles as John and I set the table to help Edna, and I put the fork upon the left and the knife upon the right and the spoon over them both with the steel bowl of the spoon right on the tip of the knife. Then we said Grace. It must be overwhelming nostalgia for teenage years of more than forty years ago; I don't know why I miss such things. But people are hard now and frightened of not being hard. If there is one single thing I miss, it is order. Without it there's clinical and every other kind of life-hating cancerous vile depression. It devours happiness and dotes on kindness to gnaw it into a cinder.

postscript

AFTER TYRANNISING ME live, my dear friend, Doctor David Gilbertson now does it by snail mail. The other day, the postman bequeathed me what appeared to be two writs typed up by the secretary from the clinic, although if you examine the top-left section of the account you learn that he toils for the Department of Psychiatry at some important university – no mean feat but then again given his extreme physical fitness he possibly runs from the university headquarters to the newest ECT intake.

Apparently an electroconvulsive treatment costs you only $118 these days – well worth the excitement, plus it's a stimulating frontal lobe conversation piece. You can say you've had it. And that's exactly right: you have.

FINAL NOTICE says the Post-It-like fluorescent adhesive sticker: legal action shall be taken. Well, I look forward to that. I'm good in court and enjoy any sort of interrogation so long as it is unfair and long. At the bottom of the urgent missive, I read that I have at least thirty days to cough up.

I'm teaching all day tomorrow at Bendigo TAFE for $255 so I'll post it from Bendigo Post Office after I'm done. As for today's events, I thought I'll be happy.